The Honey Revolution

- - -

Restoring the Health of Future Generations!

The Honey Revolution

- - -

Restoring the Health of Future Generations!

Ronald Fessenden, MD, MPH

Mike McInnes, MRPS

WorldClassEmprise, LLC

2008

The Honey Revolution

Printed in the United States of America

LCCN: 2008939688

ISBN 10: 0-9792162-1-4

ISBN 13: 978-0-9792162-1-3

Dedication and Thanks

The writing of a book seldom takes place in isolation. Several individuals and events conspired providentially, we believe, to provide motivation and encouragement for this book. When Mike McInnes from Edinburgh, Scotland first contacted hundreds of beekeepers in the United States regarding his first book, **The Hibernation Diet**, as to their interest in promoting the book through the honey industry, only a few responded. It was Jerry Brown, a third generation beekeeper from north central Kansas who seized the opportunity. He sent a copy of the book to Dr. Fessenden, his brother-in-law, to review. Dr. Fessenden found it intriguing and began an email exchange with McInnes over the science behind the claims of **The Hibernation Diet**. Within a few short months, Brown's company obtained the rights to the book and published it in the United States. Dr. Fessenden wrote an introduction. Thus began a friendship and partnership that stretched across continents.

Soon after the publication of **The Hibernation Diet** in the United States in early 2007, it became clear that a second book was needed. The accumulation of information and scientific research regarding honey was mushrooming. That information was not lost on Ron Phipps, a businessman and honey importer from New York.

In November of 2006, it was Ron Phipps, president of CPNA International, LTD who invited Dr. Fessenden to an impromptu roundtable meeting of individuals associated with the honey industry. Out of that meeting came the Committee for the Promotion of Honey and Health, Inc. It was that organization that sponsored the First International Symposium on Honey and Human Health in Sacramento, California in January of 2008. Mike McInnes was invited to be one of the presenters at that conference. Ron Phipps became so intrigued by the growing body of information regarding restorative sleep and cognitive enhancement, creative ability, and memory that he contributed to a section in this book.

To those who brought us together and gave us a platform from which to share information about nature's wonderful healthful food, this book is dedicated.

Some of the information presented at the First International Symposium on Honey and Human Health is included in this book. The authors are grateful to those many scientists and researchers who came to Sacramento to present their research findings in January 2008. However, a one day scientific Symposium could only scratch the surface of the information available from around the world. Since that event, much more has been learned that advances the health message of honey. More is being learned with each week. Still, much more needs to be discovered about the mechanisms of action of honey within the human system.

To those individuals that will take up the challenge of discovery and provide additional evidences that explain why honey is indeed a healthful food, this book is dedicated.

Finally, the subject of this writing would not be possible without the faithful and sometimes thankless work of thousands of beekeepers worldwide. The fruit of their labors brings to all of us this wonderful gift from the Creator - a miraculous natural food enjoyed by countless numbers across the centuries. Though all should be recognized for their labors, the authors would like to honor one family as representative of the many dedicated multi-generational families of beekeepers throughout the world.

To Robert and Donna Brown, second generation beekeepers, parents and in-laws of Jerry and Donette Brown, grandparents of Nathan and Britinna, all who are active beekeepers, honey producers, and wonderful examples of the best folks in the world of beekeeping, this book is dedicated.

Many sincere thanks,

Mike McInnes, MRPS
Ron Fessenden, MD, MPH
October 2008

Contents

Foreword

When **The Hibernation Diet** was first published in 2006 in the United Kingdom, it was viewed primarily as another diet book. The book was featured in multiple women's magazines and splashed across the front covers of several British tabloids as the next diet fad. Lose weight while you sleep! Who would believe it?

The US Edition of **The Hibernation Diet** published a year later added important scientific references on which the book was based. Still, the message received by most readers was that of another "easy" way to lose weight.

Unsolicited reports have come from all parts of the country and from all age groups. While many who followed the nutrition and exercise recommendations of **The Hibernation Diet** lost weight, some did not. About twenty percent of the self-reporting group lost no weight at all. Some folks lost a considerable amount of weight in a few months. Almost all who took the time to email or talk to us at conferences reported an improvement in sleep patterns. Many reported recall of vivid dreams on awakening. Some reported feeling more rested on awakening without the feelings of nausea, shakiness or headaches. Others who had trouble with interrupted sleep or short sleep patterns stated that they were sleeping through the night.

In less than a year's time since **The Hibernation Diet**'s first publication, much scientific literature has surfaced that confirms and reinforces many of the principles found in the book. The confirmation has not come in population studies that show if you eat honey at night, you will lose weight. Rather, *the research has begun to show a direct link between quality of sleep and many medical conditions and disease states.* This was one of the important messages of **The Hibernation Diet**. The book introduced us to the principles of recovery sleep and told us how to ensure getting it. The fact that one can lose weight simply by sleeping is actually a side benefit. The real benefit of following **The Hibernation Diet** was its role in what is being called *restorative sleep* and what that does for our overall health.

Eating honey before bedtime is not so much about losing weight as it is about supplying the liver with glycogen so that the brain can survive the night fast without producing adrenalin and cortisol. Chronic overproduction of these "stress hormones" may indeed be responsible for much of the morbidity and chronic disease prevalent, or rather epidemic, in our westernized cultures. Liver fueling is critical in order for restorative sleep to occur. **The Hibernation Diet** was just the beginning of the journey. In January of 2008, an international scientific Symposium sponsored by The Committee for the Promotion of Honey and Health, Inc. was held in Sacramento, California. Researchers, scientists, and physicians from nine countries around the world convened to share the results of their investigations involving honey. Several rather amazing findings were presented. Many of those findings are presented in this book along with other supportive research. We have attempted in this book to deal with as many of these issues as space allows. The research is preliminary and based on small studies. However promising these preliminary findings, there will always be skeptics who need more proof.

Honey, when consumed regularly, has a stabilizing effect on blood sugar. When compared to either sucrose or glucose alone, honey is better tolerated by those with impaired glucose metabolism or diabetes. Animal studies have shown that a diet of honey versus sucrose reduces glycohemoglobin (HbA1c) levels, the hematologic marker for glycogen that doctors use to monitor blood sugar control in diabetics. Honey may be nature's cure for the development of insulin resistance, the precursor of diabetes.

Regular consumption of honey may reduce the risk of obesity and childhood obesity. To the extent that honey may reduce oxidative stress as compared to sucrose or HFCS, its consumption may play a role in the reduction of the risks for hypertension, cardiovascular disease and other chronic metabolic conditions.

Honey may play a significant role in memory and cognitive ability. One of the presentations at the symposium presented data from a twelve month animal study that showed enhancements to memory and a reduction of anxiety in animals fed a honey-based diet compared to control groups fed sugar or an artificial sweetener.

For some readers, the technical detailed information provided in this book will be TMI - too much information. It was not our intent in writing the book to overwhelm the reader with jargon, physiology or biochemistry. However, when writing about health benefits, some degree of explanation is necessary to satisfy the skeptics. Where possible, we have included complex technical information within gray text boxes or in an appendix at the end of the book. The reader may skip these portions if desired.

We are not making *health claims* in this book! Health claims typically are associated with some regulatory agency's "stamp" of approval. Our goal is simply to present the evidence known to date. There is enough of that already to indicate that this generation's health is heading in the wrong direction. It does not take long expensive population studies to show us that the present levels of sugar and HFCS consumption are leading us toward greater prevalence of many metabolic diseases and conditions. Eliminating much of the refined sugar and HFCS from our diets and replacing it with a few tablespoons of pure honey could reverse many of the negative health trends of the past 40 years. We *are* asserting that there are many **health benefits** to be derived from consuming honey on a regular basis. These benefits are both protective and preventative. Some of the health benefits can be appreciated in days or weeks. Some will take months or years and others will take a lifetime to be fully appreciated. Our hope is that you simply get started and join us in the "honey revolution." It is a revolution with much to gain and virtually nothing to lose.

Mike McInnes, MRPS
Ron Fessenden, MD, MPH
July 2008

Introduction

This book is about honey - a wonderful, miraculous, natural food. It is not a diet book. It is a book about how regular consumption of honey will help you sleep better, provide you with better fuel for exercise, and help you achieve better health overall. This book will explain why honey is vastly superior to sugar and high fructose corn syrup (HFCS) as a source of energy. The first three chapters will describe in detail the challenges caused by 40+ years of excessive sugar and HFCS consumption and how by simply substituting honey for these sweeteners one can eliminate many of the risks associated with several metabolic conditions and diseases.

This is a revolutionary book. Revolutions are spawned out of extreme circumstances and profound need. We have a problem in America. The problem is compounding every year. More than 130 million Americans, roughly two-thirds of us, are overweight or obese. Nearly 20% of children under the age of 18 are medically obese.[1] Estimates are that by 2030, 86% of our population will be obese. Obesity and being overweight have been shown to increase the risk for developing Type 2 Diabetes, heart disease, some forms of cancer, and other disabling medical conditions. Over 24 million (8% of the population) are diagnosed with diabetes and a staggering 57 million people are pre-diabetic. Over 100,000 individuals die each year from obesity related cancers. This public health time bomb is ticking.

The total direct and indirect costs for diabetes alone, including medical costs and lost productivity, were estimated at $174 billion nationally for 2006, according to a Surgeon General's Report. As of this writing, the annual financial toll is billions of dollars more. We are heading for an epidemiologic healthcare meltdown with healthcare costs spiraling out of control. Experts agree that something has to be done, yet few can suggest viable solutions.

The problem is complex. However, the answers are surprisingly simple. Consider this - nearly every year since 1966, the per capita consumption of sweeteners has increased. This is especially true since the introduction of HFCS in the early 1970s. Since the 1980s, the per capita consumption of fructose has also increased, primarily because HFCS has slightly more fructose than does table sugar. HFCS has virtually replaced sugar as the sweetener of choice for soft drinks and most processed foods.

The published results of large population studies have indicated an association between the metabolic syndrome[2, 3] and the increased consumption of sweeteners, particularly fructose.[4, 5] The association has also been observed both in children and middle-aged adults who consumed more than one soft drink per day, regardless of whether this was a regular or diet soft drink.

This increase in incidence of the metabolic syndrome and its associated conditions of obesity, childhood obesity, diabetes mellitus, high blood pressure, and cardiovascular disease is not surprising given what we know about the metabolism of glucose and fructose in the human body. Simply put, glucose triggers an insulin spike that drives glucose into the cells where it is stored as fat. High levels of fructose consumption force the liver to metabolize it rapidly into trioses that form triglycerides, increase total cholesterol and decrease HDL cholesterol levels. It should not take expensive, elaborate population studies to convince us that the present levels of consumption of HFCS are having a disastrous yet predictable effect on the health of a nation. The results are there for all of us to see!

The HFCS, refined sugar and processed food industries have been quick to respond to published reports that indict their products. They point out that a "causal relationship" has not been proven between fructose and the host of medical conditions that have been increasing in incidence over the past 30 years. They are technically correct. Unfortunately, that is equivalent to saying that there is no casual relationship between finding open liquor containers in a wrecked car and a post mortem blood alcohol level of >0.20% (an indication of very serious intoxication) in a deceased driver at the scene of a fatal auto accident. There may be no direct proof that alcohol actually caused the fatality, but the association is quite significant, don't you think.

Large retrospective studies that have shown significant "association" between high consumption of sucrose and HFCS and the increasing incidence of metabolic diseases are not designed to prove causality! Statistically, they cannot *prove* anything. They can only show significance of association. Unfortunately, too many medical professionals, nutritionists, and public agency spokespersons have given leave of their common sense and insist on "proofs" while strong associations between dietary trends and increasing prevalence of disease continue to attack our public health!

So what about honey? If you manage to get through the first three chapters of this book, we believe that you will be convinced that honey is one possible solution to the public health challenge outlined above. Honey is certainly not part of the problem. It may take a bit of convincing that honey is not just another sweetener. After all, it is made up primarily of sugars. But what is missed with this focus on sugars is that honey contains many other miraculous principles that protect.

The state of research as of 2008 regarding honey as a healthful food is incomplete. Many of the studies that are cited throughout the book are small observational studies with fewer than 50 test subjects. Though the findings are preliminary, they are very promising.

Animal studies can lead the way in indicating physiologic responses to honey versus other sweeteners, but often, extrapolation to humans is not directly applicable due to dose and duration of exposure issues, as well as differences in species physiology. Large population studies comparing the long term physiologic effects of honey to sucrose or HFCS are expensive and difficult to carry out. Consumption of sucrose and HFCS is universal in America and most of the Western world. Identification of a control population not "exposed" to these sweeteners is virtually impossible.

One of the goals in writing this book now is to prompt additional research. Research regarding consumption of honey is necessary to confirm what we already know from history and intuition, but that will take time and money.

Perhaps, a more obtainable short-term goal in writing this book is to dispel ignorance on the part of the consuming public. However, this may be an impossible goal as evidenced by a comment made by a journalist in a recent Sunday Times. She made a few disparaging comments about honey asserting that it was "mostly sugar . . ." Tragically, there are none so prejudiced as those who are infected with the curse of "knowingness." A 1% solution of strychnine qualifies as mostly water, but has quite a different effect on the human system. The human organism is itself mostly a bag of water, but a bag of water could not build the pyramids or launch a spacecraft to the moon and return it to earth.

Here are a few of the differences between honey and refined sugars that will be discussed in more detail in the book. Honey, compared to sucrose, lowers blood glucose; honey lowers HbA1c levels (HbA1c is a marker for hyperglycemia); honey lowers triglycerides and improves HDL cholesterol; honey reduces weight gain as compared to sucrose; honey improves spatial memory and reduces anxiety; honey reduces prostaglandins/thromboxanes (both are markers for CV disease); and honey improves sleep and recovery (fat burning) physiology. Not bad for a "mostly sugar" solution.

Honey is packed, or shall we say *charged* with glucose metabolizing principles, that render this natural food anti-diabetic and give it a powerful role in fighting obesity. Honey combats oxidative stress. Honey, to some extent, can be shown to be anti-carcinogenic.

The science of honey metabolism and its application to the human system are emerging as powerful tools with which to fight disease. That honey, by its ability to optimize glucose metabolism and therefore influence and control fat metabolism, as compared to all other refined sugars or sweeteners, is of course lost on the various health professions. Equally overlooked is the principle of fueling the liver with honey before bedtime, and how that may affect sleep and recovery physiology. The consumption of honey can positively impact all the chronic adrenal driven diseases, heart disease, hypertension, Type 2 Diabetes, obesity, osteoporosis, gastric ulcers, infertility, depression, memory loss and dementias.

Honey is curative but it is not a "cure all." Honey consumption can reverse some of the indicators for diabetes. It can lower blood sugar and HbA1c levels, but only over time. It can help lower triglycerides. It will enhance immune system functioning. Honey will facilitate and insure restorative sleep. However, honey cannot fix decades of abusive dietary habits. To a generation of folks that has come to demand cures over prevention, the suggestion to substitute honey for sugar or HFCS risks being ignored by those needing immediate gratification and results. For some, this suggestion will be too late.

Honey is preventative! It is not too late for a generation of children who need desperately to change eating habits and begin eliminating the excessive quantities of refined sugar and HFCS from their diets and begin using honey. It is not too late for millions of younger and middle-aged adults to do the same and reduce their risks for a number of metabolic diseases.

Shifting momentum and changing direction in a vast dietary ocean with many competing forces at work on the "ship of public health" will not be easy. The principles presented in this book are simple. Their application over time faces many challenges not the least of which will be from our federal agencies whose recommendations and support of misguided dietary guidelines have lead us to this crisis, the processed food industry whose millions of dollars of profits are at stake, the medical associations whose research dollars and double-blinded studies have produced spurious and confounding results, and the medical professionals, nutritionists, and dietitians whose advice regarding carbohydrates and fats has done little to stymie the advance of obesity, diabetes, cardiovascular disease and other metabolic stress related conditions.

Recently I had the opportunity to spend about thirty minutes discussing the principles of this book with a curious high school teacher. She herself suffered from a few of the conditions described in the book. As she began to grasp the truth that by reducing metabolic stress simply by proper fueling of the liver with honey throughout the day and at bedtime, her interest peaked. Realizing that she could reverse over time the consequences of years of self-destructive eating behaviors, she finally exclaimed, "Why haven't we been taught these things before? Why hasn't my doctor told me about this?"

Unannounced, another recruit joined the revolution.

The Honey Revolution

Restoring the Health of Future Generations!

1 More Than Just a Sweetener, Naturally

Chapter Summary

Honey is nature's miraculous food. The nutritional composition of honey, calorie for calorie, is closer to fruit than it is to table sugar, high fructose corn syrup (HFCS) or any other sweetener. Honey contains fructose (fruit sugar) and glucose in nearly equal proportions plus other sugars and nutrients from plant nectar and pollen.

The consumption of honey has a much different effect on blood sugar in the body than sugar (sucrose) or high fructose corn syrup (HFCS) making it a unique fuel for the body's energy needs in almost every situation, awake or asleep, active or resting, well or challenged with many of life's health issues.

Honey is fuel for the brain!

Honey is sunshine energy!

Honey is Sunshine Energy

Honey is sunshine! Or more accurately, honey is a concentrated form of energy, captured from sunshine. Honey is a *fusion of light and radiant energy from the sun that reaches the earth, integrated with plant energy and then transmitted by way of nectar to honeybees who transform it into fuel for our bodies and minds - a pot of liquid gold. Honey is sunshine energy!*

Honey is a miraculous form of sunshine energy. It is distilled from sunshine by a complex, although understood, yet beguiling and numinous process known as photosynthesis, the process by which plants create a bewildering and wondrous variety of plant life, from root to stalk to leaf to flowers in their infinite variety. Plants use this sunshine energy to fund this magical process and in so doing, create pollen and sweet nectar.

A famous English song writer, Harold Baum, also a Professor of Biochemistry in his spare time, composed a lovely song about this process of photosynthesis while on the No. 22 bus between Putney Bridge and Manresa Road in London. He called it the "Photosynthesis Song" which can be sung to the tune of "Auld Lang Syne."

It begins:

> *"When sunlight bathes the chloroplast and photons are absorbed . . ."*

and concludes with these lines:

> *"the moral still is this, the one thing that keeps life alive is photosynthesis."*

The Welsh poet, Dylan Thomas, described photosynthesis as *"The force that through the green fuse drives the flower."* All green plants contain tiny little green gismos (the poet's *fuses*) called chloroplasts, which capture light energy from the sun, in the form of energized photons. As these strike the chloroplasts, this energy releases electrons.

Using this highly charged particle, the wonderful chloroplast choreographs a beautiful, botanical dance, a bio-musical reel, a molecular hoedown, an intracellular bio-ballet, during which water is split into hydrogen and oxygen, combined with carbon from atmospheric carbon dioxide to create a molecule of stored pure energy. This molecule is the monarch of all energy molecules in nature. Each molecule holds in a complex linear and/or ring structure form, six carbon atoms, six oxygen atoms, and twelve hydrogen atoms in a lovely organic, energy dense structure. This light driven vital treasury of stored energy that "keeps life alive" is what we call *glucose*, sweet glucose, one of the primary components of nectar.[6]

Flowering plants and trees produce their blossoms in a spectacular variety of colors and hues, and with an infinite diversity of arrangements and shapes. Many of these blooms are unique in their ability to create volatile fragrances, each one a symphony of mellifluous notes, precisely tuned to the olfactory senses of one particular group of pollinating insects or birds. All of this is designed to attract and guide pollinators to their sweet nectar. In exchange the flowers give up their pollen for transfer and fertilization of other plants.

The flower with its sweet nectar attracts many kinds of insects for pollination. It is only the remarkable honeybee that converts this nectar into honey, the "food of the gods" as it was known in ancient times. The honeybee, a specialized insect without which much plant life on earth would cease to exist, gathers the pollen and nectar and adds to it its own amazing contributions. Wherever we find flowering plants, we find honeybees - in every continent but one, from the Arctic Circle to the tropics to the southernmost reaches of our world. The only continent without benefit of the honeybee is the Antarctic. The honeybee takes nectar from the infinite variety of flowers available to it around the world and creates hundreds of varietals of honey, each one distinctly different in flavor and slightly different in composition. No other pollinator converts nectar into this concentrated tincture of instant energy that we call honey.

This condensed, transmuted form of light and radiant energy from the sun is food and fuel for both bees and humans. It is extremely rich in nutrients. In addition to fructose and glucose found in a near perfect 1:1 ratio, honey contains many other bioactive and protective molecules, known as antioxidants (at least 16 of them) and bioflavonoids and many other beneficially healthful substances from plants. Also contained in honey are small amounts of other sugars, amino acids, phyto-nutrients (or plant nutrients), small amounts of vitamins, organic (amino) acids, and mineral elements, plus a few enzymes added by the honeybee. When honey is consumed, the best of the nutrients obtained from the plant blossom (without the fiber or the water) is available for immediate absorption into the body for food and energy.

Composition of Honey

[Data taken from 490 samples of U.S. honey, adapted from White's chapter in *Honey*, edited by Eva Crane (London: Heinemann, 1979)]

Component	Average	Range
Water (moisture)	17.20%	12.2 – 22.9%
Fructose	38.40%	30.9 – 44.3%
Glucose	30.30%	22.9 – 40.7%
Sucrose	1.30%	0.2 – 7.6%
Maltose	7.30%	2.7 – 16%
Other sugars	1.40%	0.1 – 3.8%
Gluconic Acid	0.57%	0.17 – 1.17%
Ash	0.17%	0.02 – 1.03%
Nitrogen	0.04%	0.00 – 0.13%
pH	3.91	3.42 – 6.10%

[See Appendix A for a complete list of the active constituents of honey.]

The Sweet Golden Ratio

With very few exceptions, wherever fructose is found in nature, we find fructose *and* glucose and/or other simple sugars together in nearly equal proportions. This average and balanced ratio is found primarily in fruits and in vegetables and also *in honey*.[7] Why would this be so? The conversion of sucrose in nectar to fructose and glucose comes at a high cost. The energy demand required argues against some kind of natural or biological accident.

A philosophical explanation comes from observations in philosophy and art. We know of a Golden Ratio (*Sectio Aurea*) in art and architecture, referred to by philosophers and mathematicians Euclid, Pythagoras, Leonardo of Pisa, and Johannes Keppler. This lovely ratio refers to the relationship between the whole (object or space) to its component parts. This Golden Ratio has universal significance and is found in creation as well as in human constructs.

Is there another *Golden Ratio* that has been missed by the ancients? Could this be the perfect 1:1 ratio found in nearly all honey, the Sweet Golden Ratio, (*Sectio Aurea Dulcis*)? If so what may be the significance of this?

In 1640, an English physician, Thomas Willis remarked on the tension between what he termed the spiritual aspect of humans as opposed to the corporeal. By spirit, he referred to the mind as opposed to the corporeal body. Not only did he separate the two, he described them as in *conflict*. Modern physiology agrees with this. In fact, this tension or opposition is one of the principles outlined in **The Hibernation Diet**. By consuming a food that could fuel both mind and body simultaneously during such periods of tension, we would be able to function at our peak, physically and mentally.

This is exactly what nature has provided, thanks to the wonderful natural food provided by honeybees. ***Honey is the Sweet Golden Ratio*** of *fructose* and ***glucose*** - fructose which facilitates the uptake of glucose into the liver which in turn reserves fuel for the brain, and glucose which provides immediate fuel for muscles and every other cell in the body.

To discover why honey is the ideal fuel for human brains, it is instructive to look again at the honeybee. A study completed in the 1970s by Beckman and Chaplain provides a clue. They demonstrated that bees *in flight* provided with a glucose/fructose (fructose biphosphate) fuel learned and accomplished a task twice as fast as did bees provided only with glucose in the same concentration. It is not known whether bee brains can process fructose directly.

Honeybees are supremely intelligent insects with complex learning, olfactory, visual and navigation systems, along with advanced memory processing, by means of which they find the best, the most economic, the most energy cost effective sources of nectar. During foraging they adopt strategies incorporating distance traveled, time spent in flight, and energy-expended calculations which allow for efficient and cost effective food and energy harvesting in return for nectar gain. It seems that this 1:1 ratio of fructose to glucose in honey is as optimal for bee bio-dynamics, and for fueling both brain and locomotion demand, as it is for humans.

Honey, when used sensibly as a constituent element of a healthy eating regime will optimize the production of liver glycogen. When consumed before and during exercise, during our working day, and before rest, honey offers optimum and stress free sleep overnight (see Honey, Sleep and the "HYMN" Cycle, Poster No 14 in Appendix E). During rest, honey facilitates the release of the hormone melatonin necessary for quality sleep, and which is essential for recovery, repair, and building of new tissues, and laying down of long term memories for future retrieval.

In human modern culture we have developed a highly irrational and prejudicial view of sugar that has resulted in dangerous consumption trends. The artificial refining of cane and beet sugars which produce sucrose or table sugar and the production of high fructose corn syrup (HFCS) from corn starch introduced in large scale in the 1970s, have resulted in the annual per capita consumption of nearly 160 pounds of these sweeteners.

By comparison, the annual per capita consumption of honey is only one pound. [Contrast this with the annual per capital consumption of garlic estimated to be three and one-half pounds! Americans do not consume much honey.]

Floralflavones – The Secret Anti-sugar Signal that Bees Transmit to Us in Honey

Flavonoids are also commonly referred to as bioflavonoids. Over 5000 of them have been identified from various plants. They are commonly known for their antioxidant activity; however, the health benefits provided from these substances (specifically for cancer and heart disease) are now known to be the result of other mechanisms.

Every drop of honey, every spoon of honey, contains tiny quantities of these floral flavonoids. We call them *floralflavones*. Their names are unfamiliar to most of us: luteolin, quercetin, myricetin, kaempferol, chrysin, gallic acid, oligomeric proanthocyanidins and so on. These clever little plant molecules have been used in plant infusions for hundreds of years in China, India, Asia, Africa, and the Americas to combat a wide variety of diseases, in particular diabetes and the adrenal driven diseases discussed later in this book.

In the scientific literature these floralflavones are usually referred to as antioxidants. There are at least 16 of them found in honey at last count. Though they enter the body's cells at concentrations too low to exert any significant antioxidant benefit, this does not mean they do not have an effect in the human body. Trace amounts of these floralflavones exert powerful influences. It is a mistaken notion to believe that trace amounts of any bioactive substance are less effective than larger quantities. These compounds do not wait for the daily "minimum required dose" to be accumulated to begin their work.

These floralflavones when ingested begin work immediately to increase the antioxidant levels within cells such as increasing Vitamin C levels. They also are known to decrease capillary permeability and fragility. They

5

scavenge oxidants and free radicals and inhibit the destruction of collagen, the most abundant protein in the body. They also act as power packed anti-sugar signaling devices in the body that help control blood glucose levels. In other words, the floralflavones found in honey actually assist the body in controlling blood sugar levels. Think of it this way - *honey is nature's sweetener that combats diabetes!*

Honey, though it contains sugars (fructose and glucose and other sugars), is really nature's un-sugar!

How is it that these brilliant little active principles exert this powerful influence on blood glucose control when they are found at such microscopic levels? In a phrase, they act as molecular signals to the body's cells setting in motion a cascading series of events via activation of specific enzymes known as protein kinase enzymes.

To illustrate, these floralflavones act like the two or three sport fans that suddenly stand up during a game and in response, tens of thousands of fans in the stadium stand up and cheer. In a similar way, small concentrations of tiny bioactive molecules in our human cells can activate or signal momentous metabolic events, a molecular "wave" that circles throughout our bodies. Such is the case for floralflavones within human cells. Their concentrations in honey are miniscule, but their role in influencing glucose metabolism and other metabolic functions in the human body is huge.

We know now that many of our modern stress-related ailments are caused by chronic overproduction of cortisol. Cortisol inhibits glucose metabolism in the body and this in turn inhibits fat metabolism. When the energy pathways in any cells are inhibited and glucose and fats are not metabolized, the body (as directed by the brain) begins to degrade vital proteins in a desperate bid to maintain cell survival. This stress-activated breakdown of cellular function manifests itself as different diseases in different tissues; for example, neuro-degeneration with resultant loss of memory and other cognitive defects in brain cells, weakness in muscle tissue, and osteoporosis in bone tissue.

The good news is that our friendly floralflavones activate cell-signaling cascades in all tissues that counteract the inhibition of energy metabolism mediated by cortisol. They act at the opposite end of the energy spectrum. Honey, after its ingestion and absorption, acts at the beginning. The floralflavones found in honey act at the cellular level to improve energy metabolism and revitalize cells not functioning optimally. In other words floralflavones counteract all of the modern stress driven diseases caused by breakdown of energy metabolism, both in the body and in the mind. Our friends, the honeybees, pass on these miraculous substances to us from many floral nectars to honey.

Do honeybees themselves make use of these substances? Absolutely! Honeybees are subject to a variety of pathogenic attacks by parasites, bacteria, and viruses. The hive must be protected from such invasions. One of their main defensive strategies is the manufacture of propolis, a powerful anti-invasive substance rich in flavonoids. These flavonoids stimulate immunity in honeybees, both physiologically and within the hive. Honeybees carry immune cells known as hemocytes. There is little doubt that our wonderful floralflavones stimulate these immune cells during invasion, by similar cell signaling dynamics just as they do in our human cells.

Do they perform any other functions in bee physiology? Again the answer is an emphatic *yes*! Honeybees are very vulnerable to stress and these molecular stars are wonderful anti-stress warriors - they patrol the front line in anti-stress warfare for honeybees, just as they do for us.

We owe a huge debt of gratitude to the honeybee for passing on these miraculous substances to us by way of honey. In recent years the major drug companies have recognized the potential of these floralflavones in a variety of diseases such as Type 2 Diabetes and cancer. Millions of dollars are being spent to produce these substances artificially. Fortunately for all of us, the secret is out! Honeybees have already done the work. Floralflavones are available in honey. They do not require synthesis in a laboratory to be packaged in a pill and purchased at high cost. They can be consumed in appropriate quantities from a natural product that begins as energy from the sun, is converted into nectar and pollen by the flower, then captured by the honeybee, and delivered to us as a natural food.

This wonderful food is truly a product of:

"the force that through the green fuse drives the flower."

Or as another poet has put it:

"Honey is the soul of a field of flowers."[8]

Honey *is* more than just a sweetener. Honey is nature's soul food!

The Use of Honey in Infants

Honey is not recommended for use in infants of less than one year of age. Honey is a natural or raw food. Raw foods of any kind are not recommended for infants. The immune systems of infants younger than 12 months generally are not mature enough to deal with many kinds of antigens and other potentially harmful proteins.

Honey, like any raw food, may contain spores of the bacterium *Clostridium Botulinum*. Though botulism spores produce harmful toxins only when they grow, and they cannot grow in honey. However, it is not recommended to give honey to infants until their immune systems are mature (usually at about 12 months of age). Older children with fully developed immune systems are able to neutralize this bacterium and its potentially harmful spores. Botulism is a very serious condition in infants and attacks the nervous system, resulting in death.

Infants are no different from adults in that they require an adequate fuel store for the brain. At birth an infant is provided with a small liver glycogen store totaling around 12 grams. This is an emergency ration for the developing infant brain, in case the mother may not breast feed regularly. However, infants are not good at processing fructose as found in fruits, vegetables or honey.

This poses the question: How then is the infant brain provided for? Is there a liver fueling strategy available to infants as there is for growing children and adults?

Creation has provided another way for infants to get their brain food. It is provided for in mother's breast milk. Breast milk contains lactose. Lactose is a duo-saccharide comprised of glucose and galactose. Galactose may be likened to an infant version of fructose. Galactose is taken into the liver by virtue of the enzyme galactokinase and, like fructose, is converted to glucose, and then stored as liver glycogen. Galactose performs other very important roles in infant growth and metabolism. Infants who lack the enzyme that metabolizes galactose fail to thrive.

Honey is to children and adults as mother's milk is to infants! Both are stored in the liver as glycogen which fuel the brain.

2 The Fuels We Burn

Chapter Summary

The human body is a wonderfully complex yet efficient system. It has been designed to burn three primary types of fuels – carbohydrates, proteins or amino acids, and fats or lipids. When consumed as foods, these fuels are metabolized or broken down during the digestive process so that they can be used as sources of energy.

This chapter focuses on the metabolism of carbohydrates, specifically sucrose, a disaccharide made up of glucose and fructose; high fructose corn syrup (HFCS) which is made of glucose and fructose; and honey which is primarily glucose and fructose - three carbohydrates that are very similar with regards to sugar content. Once ingested however, honey differs remarkably from the other two.

Honey consumption (as compared to refined sugar or HFCS) leads directly to the formation of liver glycogen, thus stabilizing blood sugar levels. Honey thereby reduces metabolic stress and improves fat metabolism and disposal, thus combating two of the key parameters of the metabolic syndrome, Type 2 Diabetes and obesity.

Fats and proteins (or amino acids) are critical fuels and building blocks for human metabolism. They are essential for many processes in the body. Excess availability of fats does not influence fat utilization. While exercise releases fats into the circulation, the more intense the exercise, the smaller the percentage of fat that is burned. Fat is the primary fuel selected in the human system for rest and recovery.

Proteins or amino acids can be used by the body to create glucose to fuel the brain when liver glycogen runs low.

The Dual Fuel Storage or Energy Supply Systems of the Human Body

It is our contemporary knowledge of human physiology that gives us an example of the tensions expressed in the physiologic musings of Thomas Willis referred to in Chapter 1. As a human species, we function with essentially two distinct metabolic or fuel storage systems that seemingly coexist in tension or opposition. *One system provides energy for our muscles* during physical activity, such as when we exercise, run a marathon, work out in the gym, or walk the dog. This system utilizes primarily glucose obtained from carbohydrates absorbed through the small intestine into the circulation and driven into muscle tissue by insulin, which is released from the pancreas. Once in the muscle cell, glucose is converted to glucose-6-phosphate and later to glycogen, which stays in the cell. This glycogen is not shared with other cells. It cannot come back out of the muscle tissue to supply the energy needs of any other tissue.

The other system involves the shared glycogen store of the liver. This is the fuel supply or energy storage system for the brain. This system depends on both fructose and glucose, absorbed from the small intestine, and taken from the portal circulation into the liver where fructose facilitates the conversion of glucose into glycogen. This vital and essential energy store is not used exclusively for the brain. Glycogen stored in the liver can be released into the circulating bloodstream to provide energy for other body tissues including the heart, the kidneys, the red blood cells, and even muscles, especially at times when blood glucose runs low.

Low blood glucose levels place the brain at risk, as the brain has no capacity to store glycogen on its own. It only has a 30 second energy reserve, meaning that except for a very rapid crisis response mechanism, the brain is at risk of lapsing into a coma when blood sugar levels fall below normal.

There are two critical times when blood sugar levels can potentially fall below normal - during prolonged exercise and during sleep or the period of the night fast. During exercise, contracting muscles utilize glucose stored within the muscle cell as well as extract glucose from the circulating blood. Glucose from the circulation, most of which is released from the liver glycogen stores, is fuel required by the brain. *It is therefore perfectly correct to state that during exercise, the brain and muscles compete for the same fuel source, liver glucose.*

As muscles increase their utilization of glucose, the brain is placed at risk. As the liver store is depleted and contracting muscles increasingly use glucose, there is a very real danger of blood glucose falling below the normal acceptable range. Indeed, this occurs when athletes collapse or "hit the wall." (In the UK, they call this "The Bonk.") This is a dangerous condition and if not resolved may lead rapidly to coma.

The brain is a greedy taskmaster. It insists on being fed first, and for good reason. When we fail to provide our brain with fuel from an adequate liver glycogen reserve, or when circulating blood sugar levels approach the low range of normal or drop below normal as in hypoglycemia, the brain is forced to organize the break down of vital proteins primarily from muscle tissue. These proteins are then transported to the liver where they are converted into glucose to maintain a fuel supply for the brain. This process (known as gluconeogenesis - the creation of glucose) requires the release and activity of adrenal stress hormones, adrenaline and cortisol, and these hormones, if chronically overproduced, are behind a number of degenerative conditions associated with the modern diet.

It is important to note here that the brain does not burn fat for energy, nor does it initiate the release of stored fat from the body's cells. The human body has no mechanism for converting fat directly to glucose. Thus when the brain is in survival mode, it does not call on fat reserves for energy, but rather causes a breakdown of the body's protein to produce needed glucose. Glucose, when included in our diet from healthy foods and in the correct ratios with fructose that optimizes its uptake by the liver, may justifiably be called "*sweet* glucose" and so it is.

The brain will accept any molecule of glucose to maintain its own energy supply, regardless of the source; however, if that glucose is sourced from degraded muscle protein secondary to the repeated over-activity of the adrenal hormones, it comes at a high toll. Glucose produced from the body's own protein may turn out to be not so "sweet" at all, and indeed, over time may, in fact, become "*sour* glucose" – a biological oxymoron of a metaphor to be sure.

We humans require a reservoir of brain fuel for thinking, for mental acuity, for peak mental performance, for motivation, for focus, for learning, for formulating strategy, for challenges, for fast reactions, for passion, for drive, for inspiration, for creativity, for poetry, for music, for art, for literature, for memory processing, for dreaming, for language, for speech and consciousness, and for rest. In other words we require brain fuel for our very survival. If that was not enough, our brain requires fuel for minimizing intellectual *entropy* (loss of cerebral energy as heat).

Normal glucose metabolism is essential for proper functioning of both energy storage systems in the liver and muscles. These fuel storage systems provide critical energy for every organ in the body. It is precisely for this reason that failure of the body's finely tuned glucose metabolism mechanisms produces such widespread disastrous consequences in every system in the body, beginning with the brain.

What happens when Glucose Metabolism is Impaired

While it is not within the scope of this book to examine impaired glucose metabolism in detail, it is important to understand its causes. There are several

11

situations in which glucose metabolism in the human system becomes impaired. Impairments to glucose metabolism may either be transient (as in prolonged exercise or acute starvation) or chronic (as in a condition called insulin resistance or IR, a precursor of diabetes). Glucose metabolism impairment or the inability to metabolize glucose is the direct result of glucocorticoids (cortisol) released into the blood stream from the adrenal glands. Cortisol release is controlled by the pituitary gland in the brain. When the brain senses that glycogen stores in the liver are getting low indicating that the brain is close to running out of fuel, the pituitary gland triggers the adrenal glands to release cortisol. This is a protective mechanism, necessary for continuous functioning of the brain. Without it, brain functions would stop.

This protective action initiated by the brain comes with consequences. Cortisol inhibits the activity of insulin. Chronic and repeated release of cortisol results in a range of metabolic conditions all associated with insulin resistance (IR), a direct consequence of insulin inhibition over time. IR means that glucose, rather than being taken into the cells and metabolized as fuel or stored as glycogen, remains in the circulation as elevated levels of blood glucose. IR contributes to many conditions including obesity, diabetes, cardiovascular disease, hypertension, certain types of cancer, osteoporosis, and neuro-degenerative diseases. In addition, IR results in impaired fat metabolism, resulting in the release of increased levels of free fatty acids into the circulation.

For decades, medical science believed that the rate and availability of glucose metabolism was determined by the availability and oxidation of fatty acids. This was known as the glucose fatty acid cycle that originated from Randle in 1963.[9] The publication of a study by Robert Wolfe in 1998 changed the conventional wisdom that had been believed for decades regarding glucose and fatty acid metabolism. Wolfe demonstrated that the metabolism of fatty acids is secondary to the metabolism of glucose, rather than the reverse hypothesis that had been held for over 35 years.[10]

In other words, impairments in glucose metabolism result in impairments in fat metabolism and disposal.

Although Wolfe did not factor metabolic stress into his theory of impaired glucose metabolism, the role of cortisol and its inhibition of insulin activity had already been well established.[11]

The Effects of Chronic Metabolic Stress on the Body

Chronic metabolic stress inhibits glucose metabolism and glucose disposal in cells. This in turn results in impaired fat metabolism and disposal. The result is that both fuels - glucose and fats - now considered excess energy intake by the human system, are stored as visceral fat producing the multiple consequences of the metabolic syndrome.[12, 13, 14]

This is a critical distinction to understand. Acceptance of the fact that impaired glucose metabolism is caused by chronic metabolic stress (and the repeated excessive release of cortisol), now gives us a model for the development of Type 2 Diabetes, obesity and other related metabolic conditions. [See Poster No 12 in Appendix E for more information on this topic.]

This understanding also underscores the role for honey in combating two key conditions of the metabolic syndrome - obesity and Type 2 Diabetes - and in optimizing fat metabolism during rest.

The consumption of honey (compared to other refined sugars) reduces metabolic stress and improves fat metabolism and disposal by refueling liver glycogen and by improving glucose metabolism and disposal in peripheral cells.

The Effects of Metabolic Stress on Glucose Metabolism

Metabolic stress can be best described as a condition or set of conditions in which the body releases the glucocorticoids, adrenaline (norepinephrine) and cortisol, also known as stress hormones. Chronic excessive production of cortisol is associated with glucose intolerance, obesity and hypertension. Cortisol inhibits the activity of insulin. Over time, insulin inhibition contributes to the development of insulin resistance. Insulin resistance reduces the uptake of glucose and thus the storage of glycogen in both the liver and muscle cells resulting in elevated blood glucose levels. Insulin resistance is associated with increased risk of cardiovascular disease and other cardiovascular risk factors.[15]

Metabolic stress also contributes to impaired fat metabolism and disposal as well. Insulin resistance in fat cells reduces the effects of insulin and results in elevated hydrolysis of stored triglycerides. Increased mobilization of stored lipids in these cells elevates free fatty acids in the blood plasma.[16]

Carbohydrates

Carbohydrates are saccharides, taken from the Greek word meaning sugar. They occur as monosaccharides or simple sugars such as glucose or fructose, disaccharides such as sucrose and lactose, oligosaccharides which typically contain between two and nine monosaccharide units, and polysaccharides containing greater than ten monosaccharide units. Monosaccharides are the major source of fuel for metabolism in the body. Most carbohydrates originate from plant sources. However, lactose is the primary carbohydrate found in dairy products.

It seems a bit strange or even blasphemous in an age marked by excessive consumption of refined processed foods to state this, but *carbohydrates are not essential nutrients*. That is to say that the body can survive by getting all of its energy needs from proteins and fats. Such is hardly the case with our Western diets rich in both simple and complex carbohydrates.

Recommendations from several national and world health organizations encourage us to get anywhere from 40 to 75% of our total energy requirements from carbohydrates. These "expert" recommendations would limit the intake of simple sugars to only 10% of our energy requirements.[17, 18] Unfortunately, as we shall see later, a large percentage of our population gets upwards of 50 to 60% of its daily recommended carbohydrate supply from HFCS alone, a sweetener containing only the simple sugars fructose and glucose!

Glucose

The primary energy source for the body is glucose. As described in Chapter 1, glucose is one of the main products of photosynthesis. Most cells in the body can metabolize glucose. Glucose is critical as a building block for proteins and lipids in the body.

When consumed in large concentrations found in typical Western diets, this large glucose load causes an immediate insulin spike. This responsive and frequently excessive secretion of insulin from the pancreas rapidly drives circulating glucose into the cells. Within one and a half to two hours after a meal, little glucose remains in the bloodstream. Some glucose is metabolized for immediate energy requirements in the muscle cells, some is converted to glycogen in the liver and muscle tissue, but most is stored as fat for later use.

Then, as the blood sugar level approaches the lower end of the normal range (and sometimes falls below normal as in a "glucose crash" or hypoglycemia), or when the liver glycogen stores are depleted, the brain senses that it is running low on fuel. In other words, the brain is beginning to be "at risk." It springs into survival mode, and signals the pituitary to take immediate action. The pituitary signals the adrenal glands to release cortisol and adrenalin, powerful hormones that allow the breakdown and conversion of protein from muscle tissue into glucose.

The Glucose Paradox

In the liver, some glucose is converted to glycogen for storage and for later use by the brain, blood cells and heart muscle. However, the liver does not readily take in glucose by itself. There is at any given moment more glycogen in the liver than can be accounted for by the relatively minimal glucose absorption. This is the "glucose paradox" formulated by J. D. McGarry who theorized that most glucose gets absorbed into muscle cells where it is converted into lactic acid in the anaerobic metabolic cycle. This is true especially in situations of energy depletion during exercise. The lactic acid is then taken to the liver where it is converted into the building blocks that form liver glycogen. Much of the body's liver glycogen is produced indirectly from lactic acid rather than directly from glucose in the blood.

Fructose and the Fructose Paradox

Fructose cannot be metabolized directly by most human cells. Whereas every cell in the body can metabolize glucose, it is the liver that is the primary location for fructose metabolism. When fructose is ingested by itself, it is rapidly converted to trioses that enter the fatty acid cycle to form triglycerides. In Chapter 3 more of the challenges presented by fructose will be discussed.

When fructose and glucose are ingested together in nature's perfect ratio - *that is another story*. When honey, containing both fructose and glucose, is consumed, something entirely different takes place. Fructose, it seems, has a sublime trick up its molecular sleeve. It *regulates* glucose intake into the liver. In chemical or metabolic terms, fructose serves as an accelerator for glucose conversion to glycogen. In other words, it facilitates conversion of glucose to glycogen in the liver. This wonderful trick we call the ***Fructose Paradox***.

This is how it works. Fructose first enters the liver cell with the assistance of fructokinase. Once in the liver cell, fructose liberates the glucose enzyme, glucokinase, an enzyme that is locked up in the liver cell nuclei. Glucokinase optimizes and regulates glucose uptake into the liver. In the liver, glucose is converted to and stored as glycogen. In other words fructose optimizes glucose uptake into the liver, and this in turn regulates blood glucose stability. It does this by preventing a large glucose load from entering the circulation. Thus, honey with its near equal portions of fructose and glucose (similar to most fruits and vegetables) is an ideal natural form of energy for replenishing liver glycogen.

As the liver is the only organ in the body able to take in and digest fructose, fructose can be characterized as the quintessential brain food or fuel, both because of its regulating glucose uptake into the liver and by itself being converted to glucose in the liver.

As we will see in more detail in Chapter 3, there appear to be distinct differences between the rate of formation of liver glycogen, the insulin response, and the resultant blood sugar levels when glucose and fructose contained in honey are ingested versus glucose and fructose as metabolized from sucrose or as found in HFCS.

Glucokinase – the Glucose Enzyme

Glucokinase is found in four different areas in the human body. The glucokinase in each location plays a critical role in the regulation of glucose metabolism in the body. *The primarily location for glucokinase is in the nucleus of hepatocyte - the human liver cell.* Other locations where glucokinase is found are in the pancreas, the hypothalamus of the brain and in certain cells of the small intestine. The glucokinase in these areas works in a regulatory manner allowing the cells in these organs to respond to rising or falling levels of blood glucose. Glucokinase activity can be amplified or reduced in minutes by actions of the glucokinase regulatory protein (GKRP), influenced by the presence or absence of very small amounts of glucose and fructose.

Thus, the presence of very small amounts of fructose *accelerates* the release of glucokinase (GK) by the action of glucokinase regulatory protein (GKRP). This sensitivity to fructose allows GKRP and GK to act as a "fructose sensing system" which signals that a mixed carbohydrate meal is being digested and accelerates the utilization of glucose into glycogen. Once the liver hepatocytes are replete with glycogen, excess glucose is converted into triglycerides and stored as fat. Glucokinase activity in the cytoplasm rises and falls dependent on the available glucose.

Glycogen

Glycogen is a polysaccharide made up of multiple molecules of glucose. The average adult liver can store between 75 - 100 grams of glycogen. Glycogen can also be stored in muscle tissue. However once glycogen is stored in muscle tissue, it stays there to be used exclusively by muscle cells. Only the glycogen stored in the liver is accessible to other organs. Glycogen stored in the liver is the primary fuel reservoir for the brain.

Fats - the Body's Essential Building Blocks

There are other vital building blocks of life, used not just for energy, but also for all the repair and maintenance work required by our bodies. Fats or lipids are such essential building blocks. Somewhere around the early 1950s, fats, especially what are called saturated fats, began to have a bad reputation as a necessary fuel for life.

For decades, the American Heart Association, the American Dietetic Association, the American Medical Association, the National Cholesterol Education Program (NCEP), the U.S. government and others supported by the corn, wheat, and highly profitable processed food industries have repeated the warning "beware of saturated fats." This message persists in spite of the fact that the connection between saturated fat in the diet and elevated cholesterol has never really been made. As Dr. Atkins points out in Chapter 1 of his book, [19] it was Dr. William Castelli, the original director of the Framingham Heart Study, who revealed the shocking inside story on Framingham in 1992: "the people with the lowest serum cholesterol were the ones who ate the most saturated fat and cholesterol and took in the most calories." This admission is hardly a blanket condemnation of dietary fats.[20] Could it be that something else is the culprit? Logic and common sense would argue that there is.

As the amount of fat consumption has decreased over the past three to four decades, *the amount of sugar and HFCS consumption has increased.* The food industry quickly discovered just how easy it was to make low fat foods taste good. Just add sugar or HFCS. Low fat, high carbohydrate diets have proliferated producing a population plagued with obesity, diabetes, and increasing cardiovascular disease. This is due in large measure to overwhelming misinformation from many sources including bad science, nutritionists and medical organizations which should have known better, the processed food industry with its huge marketing budgets, and the federal government and its agencies.

Beginning in the 70s, the manufacture of HFCS from cornstarch made this the sweetener of choice for processed foods, especially soft drinks. It is no coincidence that for the past 35+ years, we have witnessed a pandemic of obesity, childhood obesity, and an increase in the incidence of diabetes, cardiovascular disease, obesity-related cancers and neuro-degenerative diseases such as Alzheimer's disease and Parkinsonism.

Fats Are Essential for Life

Fats are vital to our metabolic life. We humans have a well recognized fat hunger and for good reason. We ignore this requirement for fat at our peril. To demonstrate just how important fats are, animal studies have shown that feeding fats directly into the liver reduces nerve feedback signals relating to liver energy status by way of the vagus nerve to the brain. When fat metabolism is blocked, the liver energy status is lowered and nerve signals activate appetite and food seeking activities.[21]

Fats also play a vital function in our immune systems. They work as signaling molecules and as the foundation for vital transmitters, known as prostaglandins.[22] It is not within the scope of this book to examine fats in great detail, but it is vital to understand that the focus on the harmful effects of excess fat storage in our modern metabolic life should not blind us to the critical and beneficial roles that fats play in our overall health.

Fats as Fuel

There are two fundamentally different fat storage depots that are used during rest and during exercise. Muscle cells use their fat storing facility to stockpile fats as triglycerides. This fat store is used exclusively during exercise, as the muscle cell contracts. The other fat stores are spread around the body in obvious subcutaneous locations at the waist and hips and in not so obvious locations as the visceral fat stores around the organs in the abdomen. The fat stored in these various locations is known as adipose tissue or fat.

Adipose fat is used for energy requirements both during rest and during exercise. During exercise, contracting muscles can use both the muscle fat stored as triglycerides in muscle cells and fats stored as adipose tissue from around the body. Adipose fats are brought to muscle cells by the circulating blood. Exercise releases fatty acids into the circulation. One would conclude that this release of fats is in direct response to exercise demands. Intuitively, it would appear that the availability of fat would relate to the amount of fat burned.

Fat Availability versus Fat Utilization

Surprisingly there is no connection between the quantity of fats released from body adipose stores and the amount of fat used in contracting muscles. In other words, there is no direct relation between availability of fat and the oxidation or metabolism of fats. One would think that availability would control or somehow relate to utilization. However, this is not the case.

This is a very important distinction and overturns one of the most enduring myths prevalent throughout sport - both recreational and professional - that releasing fats from fat stores results in an increased utilization of fat.

Many recreational athletes, who train with the prospect of burning extra fat, imagine that exercising and not eating will result in the oxidization of more fat. Labels and placards on some of the equipment on which athletes train attempt to make this myth credible. Many of us have jumped on a treadmill or cross-trainer and selected the "Fat Burning" mode or targeted our heart rate within the "Fat Burning Zone" believing that we were increasing our fat burning by this activity. *Nothing could be further from the truth.*

The quantity of fat used during any exercise protocol depends *only* on the level of intensity of exercise in inverse proportion to the intensity, and not on the level of fats released from stores into the bloodstream. A study by Professor Robert Wolfe of Texas University, demonstrated that an increase of fats in the bloodstream by a factor of 20 had no effect on the quantity of fat metabolized.[23] In fact, *the more intense the level of exercise, the less fat we burn as a percentage of metabolic requirements.* At peak aerobic exercise levels, only 10% of our energy requirements come from fat.

What happens then to the circulating fats released during exercise and not taken up and used by contracting muscle cells? They are returned to the fat stores (adipose tissue and muscle stores) in the post exercise period. In fact, as much as 90% of these circulating fats may be returned to fat stores following exercise. During an exercise protocol, as much as 25% of circulating fats are returned to fat stores.[24]

As a marathon runner in the 70s, the author remembers training with a respected cardiologist. He encouraged those attending a marathon training symposium to use caffeine before a race to liberate free fatty acids as fuel for the long haul to boost endurance. However, taking a thermogenic drug such as caffeine or even a more powerful drug such as ephedrine that will release extra fats during exercise is totally counter productive. Most of the circulating fats are simply returned to fat stores. Some will be left adhering to blood vessel walls in the post-exercise period as insulin is released. In addition, ephedrine is a catecholamine type compound and will place increased stress on the cardiovascular system. Generally, the outcome of trying to increase circulating fats during exercise is that the exerciser is adding to the risk of atherosclerosis and cardiovascular events further down the line.

The Effect of Training on Fat Burning

Some of the confusion around this question arises from references in sports literature that state that exercise training increases the amount of fat used during any exercise protocol relative to the amount of carbohydrate (glucose) consumed. This is factually correct. Any trained athlete will use more fat relative to carbohydrate in the same exercise protocol, compared to an untrained athlete.

However, on any given day for that trained athlete, the overall rule prevails. The relative quantities of glucose to fats consumed will be determined by the level of intensity of exercise, and may not be altered by increasing the quantity of circulating fats.[25] The effect of exercise intensity has the force of a universal law of nature and seems to prevail over all locomotive species, whatever their individual exercise capacities, and in all environments, including at sea level and at altitude where parameters may be expected to differ significantly.[26]

Obesity and Fatigue – the Fuel Conundrum When More Is Less

Fatigue is one of the most widely reported complaints given by patients to their physicians. Since the majority (64%) of the population is overweight or obese, this appears to be a contradiction. Each overweight individual carries a large energy store in the form of stored body fat or adipose tissue. Thus there is available to this individual at any time of the day or night a vast reservoir of spare energy, which may be released to meet energy requirements and used to improve energy status. Because of this, one could conclude that this energy reserve would therefore serve to reduce fatigue. That this does not occur, i.e., the great majority of overweight or obese individuals suffer from forms of energy inertia and chronic fatigue, highlights one of the enduring contradictions in human energy metabolism.

During recovery and to some degree during exercise, fats from muscle tissue and from adipose stores may be used to meet the energy requirements of all organs and systems of the body except for one. The brain is that one exception. The brain cannot metabolize fats for energy at any time.

Mental fatigue (myasthenia) is one of the most debilitating forms of energy fatigue. During lengthy periods of concentrated effort when no physical activity is undertaken, the body's excess energy store of fat is not available for use by the brain. Neither can fats be converted to glucose or glycogen, the primary fuel used in brain (neural) cells. It is ironic that given an excess of fuel stores available to a majority of individuals, this reserve is not available to meet the energy demands brought on by either physical or mental fatigue, except in one near terminal situation.

Ketosis, the Second Stage of Starvation

Brain cells and other nerve cells may use fats as fuel in one very special circumstance and that is during starvation. In humans, the first few days of famine are characterized by the metabolism of protein to maintain fuel supply to the brain. This is similar to the physiologic state functioning both during exercise and during the night fast when low liver glycogen levels force the brain to activate stress hormone release. This hormone, cortisol, degrades muscle proteins which are carried to the liver in the form of amino acids and transformed into glucose so that there is available and adequate fuel reserve for the brain.

However, this type of physiology is abandoned after a few days in favor of another known as ketosis. Ketosis is a situation produced when fats are transferred to the liver and converted into ketones, small four-carbon fat molecules that may be used in the brain.

This second stage phase of starvation is interesting because ketones do not require the continued degradation of muscle proteins to create new glucose; therefore, there is no requirement for release of adrenal hormones with all the ill effects that they may bring. In this unique type of physiology, brain function is well maintained. In this case, fats, in the form of ketones, may be used to provide energy in brain cells. For an obese individual who is provided with an adequate supply of water and all other essential nutrients, this type of strategy may be maintained for several months as a form of weight loss.

Atkins, Benign Dietary Ketosis, Migratory Birds and Hibernating Animals

Essentially this was the type of approach use by Atkins in his book, Dr. Atkins' *New Diet Revolution*.[27] Although Atkins' dietary recommendations are a valid approach to forcing fat metabolism, they are difficult for many to sustain, except for those whose dietary intake is under direct medical supervision.

Atkins focused on a fundamental ability of our human physiology to activate benign ketosis, a strategy also used by migrating birds and hibernating animals. Migrating birds, for instance, may double their weight in a two-week period prior to migration. Essentially their entire energy intake during this pre-flight period is converted to fat stores with the exception of a small liver glycogen reserve. This liver glycogen reserve is used only during takeoff to create the power required to overcome gravity and energize flight. Then these amazing creatures switch their metabolic energy use to fats for powering wing muscles, and ketones to maintain energy supply to the brain necessary for navigation. If the birds miscalculate distance, time, fuel to output ratio, or perhaps run into adverse weather conditions and are blown off course, they may run low on fat stores. The result is serious metabolic trouble and perhaps fatal consequences.

Low energy stores will trigger the degradation of proteins. These proteins will come from gut and muscle proteins. (This pending energy crisis situation is similar to what happens to humans during exercise and during the night fast if our livers are not well stocked with glycogen.) These migratory birds are now in a chronic state of adrenal overdrive. If they are unable to find a suitable landing area for rest and refueling, they will soon fall out of the sky. Many studies on migrating birds demonstrate that if their fat stores remain adequate, they will avoid the state of raised metabolic stress.[28]

Hibernating animals share a similar metabolic dependence on fats. However, their ability to survive depends on their ability to reduce their metabolic rate and suspend certain physiologic functions. Given a safe environment and good stores of reserve fat, they can last through the winter without incurring metabolic stress.

Humans on the other hand have no such sustained mechanism for avoiding metabolic stress when their liver glycogen stores are depleted. Even during the second stages of starvation, the ability of human metabolism to utilize ketones from fats is difficult to sustain indefinitely.

Carbs for Rest and Fats for Exercise - a Metabolic Fantasy

During rest periods, the human body utilizes mostly fats as fuel. This statement overturns another of the most prevalent myths surrounding human metabolism - that the primary fuel for exercise is fat and the primary fuel for rest is glucose. It is profoundly counter-intuitive to accept the fact that we burn more fat during rest than we do during exercise. The partition and selection of fuels during both rest and exercise is overlooked by most health professionals and by most sport coaches and athletes, the very groups who should be aware of this important information.

To illustrate, let us suppose that the popular view is correct - that fats are the fuel selected for exercise, and glucose is the fuel used during rest. There are four essential fuel stores in the body - liver and muscle glycogen, and body (adipose) fat and muscle fat. To further illustrate, let us select as a test subject an individual who is overweight, one who does no physical exercise. His sluggish metabolism may be assumed to require about 2500 Calories over a 24-hour period. From where would these calories be sourced?

According to the popular "theory," resting metabolism utilizes only glucose and not fat for required metabolic needs (remember our subject does not exercise). The source of energy for this individual, therefore, would have to be exclusively from liver glycogen as muscle glucose is not shared with other tissues or cells. Therefore, this means that every calorie required for rest must be sourced from the liver. The liver is the only glycogen store able to supply all other organs and tissues with glucose in the postprandial period (the period after a meal). Over 24 hours the liver must provide some 2500 Calories or 625 grams of glucose in the form of glycogen.[29] Given a liver capacity of only 75 grams, our subject would have to eat more than eight meals over the 24-hour cycle to provide the liver with enough glycogen to fuel his resting metabolism. His diet would have to be of substance and quantity that could be converted directly to glycogen in the liver – no protein or fat.

This is obviously not the way humans eat. We are omnivores consuming a mix of carbohydrates, proteins and fats from plant and animal sources. If our subject followed the recommendations of national and world health organizations and consumed about half of his caloric needs from carbohydrates, he would now need to consume 16 meals in 24 hours to keep his liver supplied with glycogen. However, only one-third of the available carbohydrate from any meal will be converted to glycogen in the liver. Our insatiable subject would now require some 48 meals over the 24-hour period to keep his liver stocked. Unfortunately while providing sufficient resources to meet all the metabolic energy requirements of a 24-hour period in such a resting individual, he now is growing even more obese from the fats and excess carbohydrates not incorporated into liver glycogen.

To follow this twisted logic, such an individual would require up to 16 efforts to refuel the liver during each 8-hour rest period at night. Without this, the liver glycogen store would be depleted, blood glucose would fall and remain below normal. Coma would follow and death would be the likely outcome.

Our illustration has moved from the ridiculous to the surreal just to highlight one simple metabolic truth - *fat is essentially selected in human metabolism as the fuel for rest and recovery.* Glucose is primarily the fuel to power exercise and locomotion.

We are not claiming here that glucose is not used as fuel during rest. It is, but it is primarily utilized as fuel for the brain. This is one of the key principles elaborated in this book. Neither are we claiming that fats are not used during exercise. They are, but the quantity is not significant. In fact, the higher the intensity of exercise, the lower the amount of fat burned.

We hope that the reader will forgive this above excursion into the bizarre realm of metabolic fantasy. It could have been omitted entirely but for the fact that the myth about fats as a primary fuel for exercise is encountered on a daily basis, being universally repeated in gyms, clinics and on playing fields across the entire western world.

The mistaken notion that fats are not used as energy during rest should encourage those who hold this view to focus on refueling the small critical liver glycogen store before bed. Instead, the myth that "one should not eat before bed as the food will only turn to fat" continues to be believed even by medical professionals.[30] Couple that myth with another popular myth - that exercise burns fat, not glucose - and one ends up with two mutually contradictory myths in a kind of surreal metabolic doublet.

This would be amusing if it were not for the realization that such myths reinforce the thinking of the great bulk of our population regarding going to bed with a depleted liver. They retire late, three or four hours after an early evening meal, and are awakened by the release of adrenalin and cortisol that results from a liver depleted of necessary glycogen in the early morning hours. The demands of the brain for glycogen may activate stress physiology every night of the week, for weeks, months and years, with the result being an increasing tide of adrenal driven diseases characterized in medicine as the metabolic syndrome. These myths are not only a specious form of metabolic fantasy, they are profoundly dangerous and play a significant role in contributing to modern metabolic malfunction.

Locomotion versus Sleep and the Body's Energy Status Gage

Two very different physiological activities – locomotion and hunger - are fundamental, essential components of human physiology. One is active, the other is regulatory. Locomotion (the activity of food seeking and/or exercise in general) and hunger (which is a very effective energy status gage) are coupled in a small region of the brain known as the suprachiasmatic nucleus (SCN) of the hypothalamus. It is the function of the SCN to anticipate the energy requirements of locomotion and monitor the energy status of the liver in order to insure adequate fuel supply for the brain during these periods. Hunger is the conscious sensation resulting from the subconscious activity of the energy status indicator in the SCN.

The key to normal physiologic activity of both locomotion and hunger is, of course, the liver. If the liver glycogen stores remain adequate, the brain functions normally during prolonged periods of locomotion. Metabolic stress, brought on by the release of cortisol on signal from the SCN when liver glycogen is low, is avoided.

A correlate of this locomotion/hunger couplet is another pair of physiologic activities - sleep and energy status. Sleep, similarly to locomotion is an energy driven process meaning that during rest, fuel for the brain (glycogen) must be dispersed from the liver. Again it is the energy status gage in the SCN that closely monitors the energy availability and reacts when the fuel level falls low. If the liver is not stocked with glycogen, recovery physiology is compromised and fat-burning during rest is not optimized. Stress hormones will be activated and the resultant metabolic stress will inhibit both glucose and fat metabolism. By eating before bed, we ensure adequate liver glycogen to fuel the brain for the night fast, and allow recovery physiology to burn fat. [More information on this topic is included in Chapter 5.]

Both locomotion (exercise) and sleep are similar in one regard. Energy requirements for both are monitored and regulated in the SCN, which functions as the body's energy status gage. Adequate liver glycogen stores are essential for both exercise and sleep. Without adequate liver glycogen, metabolic stress is initiated.

A Brief Word about Proteins or Amino Acids

Dietary sources of protein are eggs, meat, dairy products and legumes. Proteins are digested by enzymes in the stomach into polypeptides which supply over twenty amino acids used by our systems. Nine of these amino acids (also called "essential amino acids") cannot be synthesized by our bodies and must come from these dietary sources. Amino acids are used to synthesize other proteins (or chains of amino acids) which are the basic building blocks for the body, its RNA templates, and the multiple regulatory proteins required by our systems. Amino acids can also be directly utilized as fuel for the body by oxidation either by the urea or citric acid cycles. The liver is the primary organ in the body that metabolizes protein by converting it to glucose (gluconeogenesis). Proteins, like carbohydrates, provide the body with four Calories per gram of food energy.

During exercise, proteins can be used as back-up fuel for the brain as the liver becomes depleted of glycogen. However, the use of protein in this circumstance is expensive in terms of overall energy toll and can be easily avoided by refueling the liver. This physiologic process (the degrading of muscle and transfer of amino acids to the liver for conversion to glucose) is a normal and essential part of human metabolism. This process means that the carbon atoms and energy held in the amino acids are not lost or wasted but recycled and used as energy substrates. However, the benefits of this type of metabolic conservation are lost in situations where this process is excessive as it may be during prolonged exercise or during the night fast when and if liver glycogen stores run low.

In particular, this is the case in western society where we are instructed by misinformed diet gurus to avoid eating late in the evening or just before bedtime. As stated earlier, there is not a shred of scientific evidence to support this ill-founded prohibition. Nevertheless it is frequently repeated in the media. In reality, this advice can be blamed for contributing to the increasing tide of adrenal driven, metabolic stress related diseases, including diabetes, heart disease and obesity.

3 Differentiating Honey from Other Sweeteners

Chapter Summary

Honey is primarily a carbohydrate made up of fructose and glucose in ratios similar to the 1:1 ratio of fructose to glucose found in sucrose and the 55:45 ratio of fructose to glucose found in HFCS 55. However, observational data obtained from human and animal studies indicate that something truly remarkable occurs after ingestion of honey that allows us to differentiate it from these other sweeteners.

The consumption of honey as compared to the consumption of sucrose or HFCS results in:

- A lower insulin response and lower blood glucose levels lower HA1c levels,
- Higher levels of HDL cholesterol (the "good cholesterol"),
- Lower triglycerides,
- Increased fat metabolism at rest, and
- Reduced intracellular oxidative stress.

The reasons for these remarkable differences, especially in individuals with impaired glucose metabolism, though not entirely understood, have been confirmed in multiple observational studies in animals and humans.

For centuries honey has enjoyed a positive image as nature's sweet substance. Biblical references refer to its sweetness. Culinary schools and chefs consider it an alternative to sugar in cooking and baking. Grocery stores and health food outlets stock it on the "sweetener" shelves or next to the syrups. To most people, honey is simply one sweetener in a market flooded with sweeteners and sugar substitutes.

A significant message is missed and a great disservice done to this natural product when one considers honey only as a "sweetener." To be sure, honey is sweet. But honey is more than just a sweetener. It is a wonderful, natural, historic food containing secrets that have been hidden or ignored for too long in the United States. Honey is what the marketing industry refers to as a "functional food," also known as a nutraceutical - a natural food that delivers a health benefit. The past ten years have witnessed an emergence of a major marketing trend focusing on these foods. The impact of these marketing trends on consumption has been impressive for foods such as tea, almonds, brown rice, dark chocolate, tomatoes, dairy products, and eggs.

The success of these marketing campaigns is due not just to slick advertising, though that plays a big part. Behind the campaigns is solid scientific research uncovering what many natural food enthusiasts (and mothers and grandmothers) have known for decades. Certain natural foods are beneficial because they contain nutrients not found in processed foods and refined sugars. These nutrients are responsible for numerous healthful benefits, including, just to name a few, lowering of blood pressure, reductions in triglycerides and cholesterol, reductions in the risk of cardiovascular disease and some forms of cancer, improvements in the immune system, and regulation of blood sugar.

Though the consumption of honey has been associated with positive healthful dietary habits for centuries, mentioning honey and health in the same phrase seems to defy conventional wisdom today. This may be because honey is only thought of as a sweetener. The negative association of sweets with obesity, diabetes, tooth decay and other metabolic conditions has cast a wide shadow over many otherwise healthful natural foods including honey.

The challenge for honey is no more clearly put than to note that since the early 1970s, the consumption of honey in the United States has been linked directly to the consumption of other sweeteners. As public health concerns (and there are many) focus on the association of increased consumption of sucrose (refined table sugar) and high fructose corn syrup (HFCS) driving demand and consumption of these products down, the consumption of honey is sure to decrease in a parallel fashion.

This need not be the case, especially since the annual per capita consumption of honey is now only about one pound. Education of the consuming public is essential to insure continued increases in honey demand and consumption while the consumption of sucrose and HFCS is reduced. Honey is a sweet carbohydrate to be sure. However, it is essential to differentiate it from sucrose, HFCS and other so-called artificial sweeteners.

At first blush, this is a formidable challenge. Honey is made up primarily of glucose and fructose in a nearly equal ratio. Sucrose is also equal portions of glucose and fructose joined as a disaccharide until separated by the digestive process by enzymes in the stomach. HFCS 55 and HFCS 42 (the most commonly used blends of HFCS) have ratios of 55:45 and 42:58 fructose to glucose respectively. On the surface, we have three sugary substances, all nearly equal in their composition of glucose and fructose, yet uniquely different with regard to their effects within the human system.

Observations that Differentiate Honey, Sucrose, and HFCS

In order to differentiate between honey, sucrose, and HFCS, we will first observe and compare the measured results of ingesting these three carbohydrates that appear to be very similar with regard to their primary sugar content. Later we will explain some of the possible mechanisms by which human metabolism differentiates between them.

Honey is made up of approximately 40% fructose (with a range from 31 to 44%) and 40% glucose (with a range from 23 to 41%) depending on varietals. The differences in fructose to glucose ratios in honey are explained by the variable sucrose content of nectars upon which the honeybees forage. After consumption of honey, the individual molecules of glucose and fructose pass through the stomach and are rapidly absorbed in the duodenum and small intestine by way of transport mechanisms described later.

Short-term animal studies have indicated that rats fed honey gain less weight, have lower blood sugar levels, lower levels of triglycerides and higher HDL cholesterol levels versus rats fed a diet of sucrose.[31] When similar quantities of ingested honey are compared with glucose and sucrose as to their effect on blood sugar levels in humans, again honey comes out ahead.[32, 33]

Honey's Role in Regulating Blood Sugar

Regular consumption of honey can help to regulate blood glucose. On the surface, this proposition seems rather counter intuitive, sort of like eating bacon to control your cholesterol. But is it so far fetched? Preliminary clinical scientific evidence would indicate that it is not.

Several studies have shown that blood sugar responses to the ingestion of honey, sucrose and glucose are remarkably different. Blood sugar levels measured at 60 and 90 minutes after ingestion of comparable amounts of honey, sucrose and glucose indicate a significantly lower level of measurable blood sugar from honey than from either sucrose or glucose.[34] And in fact, the more impaired one's glucose tolerance happens to be, the better one's tolerance for honey.[35] In other words, the more glucose intolerant one is, the lower the blood sugar response after honey ingestion versus the higher the blood sugar response after consuming sucrose or glucose. The differences in blood sugar responses are magnified even more in Type 2 and Type 1 diabetics in whom glucose intolerance is more advanced.

One of the reasons for honey's remarkable regulatory ability was described in Chapter 2 as the Fructose Paradox. The near one-to-one ratio of fructose to glucose found in honey - nature's perfect ratio - actually *facilitates* glucose intake into the liver. Fructose optimizes the conversion of glucose to glycogen in the liver by prompting the release of glucokinase from the liver nuclei. Glucokinase converts glucose to glycogen, which is then stored in the liver. Thus a large glucose load is prevented from entering the circulation and causing a sharp elevation of blood sugar. Consuming natural energy-packed honey with its ideal ratio of fructose and glucose is an ideal way to replenish liver glycogen and at the same time control blood glucose levels.

No other sugar or combination of sugars possesses this ability. But there is another and perhaps even more powerful "regulatory" role for honey. *Consuming honey can actually increase the metabolism of fat during rest.* By replenishing liver glycogen and by improving glucose metabolism and disposal in peripheral cells, honey consumption (compared to other refined sugars) reduces metabolic stress and improves fat metabolism and disposal, thus combating two of the key parameters of the metabolic syndrome, obesity and Type 2 Diabetes.

In Chapter 5 we will describe in more detail the role of honey when consumed before bedtime in optimizing fat burning during rest. This principle is based on the fact that an adequate supply of glucose or liver glycogen during the night fast assures fatty acid metabolism during recovery periods. When there is inadequate liver glycogen for the brain during sleep, cortisol release interrupts fat metabolism and limits the amount of fats being burned for energy. [See Appendix E, Poster No 12 for a more technical explanation of how glucose (glycogen) availability controls fatty acid oxidation.]

> *Given the fact that honey performs a significant and valuable role in "regulating" blood glucose thereby reducing metabolic stress and improving fat metabolism and disposal, the lifelong health benefits from consuming honey rather than sugar or HFCS, are amazing. The substitution of small amounts of honey for the current consumption of large amounts of sugar or HFCS could reap enormous individual and public health consequences. Prevention of metabolic stress by eating honey may be the miracle cure for many of the next generation's stress-related diseases and conditions.*

Honey and Reduction of Intracellular Oxidative Stress

We know that prolonged high blood glucose levels as the result of impaired glucose metabolism, insulin resistance, or diabetes, contribute to oxidative stress within the cells throughout the body. Damage caused by oxygen free radicals occurs to protein and lipids, especially in the membranes of cells and to the DNA of the cell nuclei.[36] All cells in the body are susceptible to this damage caused by these free radicals, particularly those cells that are found in neural or brain tissue. It is the unique makeup of neuronal tissue with its high levels of fatty acids in their membranes and high oxygen requirements that contributes to the production of higher levels of free radicals.

Hyperglycemia or chronic high blood sugar levels eventually cause irreversible damage to the brain through this increase in free radical generation. This brain cell damage is the direct result of impaired glucose metabolism combined with decreasing antioxidant production in the body as we age. Honey consumption will lower glucose levels, reduce the risk of impaired glucose metabolism, *plus* provide small amounts of antioxidants necessary to reverse the effects of free radicals on the aging brain and nervous system.

The link between early onset Type 2 Diabetes and an increased risk for dementias and cognitive decline and impairment has been demonstrated.[37] Several studies have shown that poor glycemic control or impaired glucose tolerance has a significant impact on working memory, verbal declarative memory and brain processing speed or executive functions.[38, 39] The earlier one achieves and maintains good glycemic control, the smaller the impact of diabetes on cognitive functions above the age of 70. This observation from Awad and Messier[40] argues for the elimination of much of the sugar and HFCS consumed from an early age and the substitution of honey as a way of preventing a decline in cognitive ability, memory and reducing the risk of vascular dementia or Alzheimer's disease.

Atherosclerosis and heart disease are also associated with Type 2 Diabetes. The detrimental effects of chronically impaired glucose metabolism associated with complications of cerebrovascular disease[41] also have a disastrous impact on blood vessels of the heart and throughout the body. Elevated levels of the amino acid homocysteine (HCY), a condition known as hyperhomocysteinemia, are also associated with an increased risk of heart disease, osteoporosis and Alzheimer's disease, presumably due to the effects of oxidative damage.

Prevention of oxidative damage associated with the several complications of diabetes and the progression of other age related disorders including cancers, mitochondrial dysfunction, chronic inflammation, autoimmune diseases is more easily accomplished than is treatment. Lifelong excessive consumption of sugar and HFCS is known to be associated with all of these conditions.

The regular consumption of honey, because of its ability to regulate blood sugar by lowering circulating blood sugar levels and to reduce intracellular oxidative stress, seems to be a sweet simple solution that will reduce the risks of developing these diseases.

In Chapter 8, several stunning examples are provided that illustrate the preventive and protective effects one gains simply by consuming honey. The physiologic effects provided from eating honey are not available from the consumption of other refined sugars such as sucrose and high fructose corn syrup.

Honey Protects against Elevated Triglycerides from Fructose

In the section on fructose that follows on page 33, we will see that fructose, a monosaccharide whose consumption has increased steadily since the 1970s, actually contributes to the elevation of triglycerides in the body. Yet if the source of fructose is honey, which contains fructose and glucose in nearly equal proportions, the same hypertriglyceridemic (elevated serum triglycerides) effect is not observed.[42] This is an amazing distinction that clearly differentiates honey from HFCS or sugar and other starches.

This study demolishes the notion that because honey contains fructose, it must therefore express the same pro-oxidative effect and result in elevated circulating triglyceride levels as known to occur with a diet high in fructose (as in HFCS). Honey-fed rats showed lower levels of triglycerides and lowered pro-oxidant effects than those fed starch or HFCS. Additional human studies are required to identify mechanisms responsible for this effect. [For more information on this subject, see Poster No 2 in Appendix E.]

Sucrose

Sucrose or refined table sugar is a disaccharide made up of equal parts of fructose and glucose. In humans, sucrose is very readily digested in the stomach into its component sugars, by acidic hydrolysis. In other words, the acid content of the stomach allows an enzyme, glycoside hydrolase, to catalyze the digestion of sucrose into separate monosaccharides glucose and fructose. Glucose and fructose are rapidly absorbed into the bloodstream in the small intestine. Some amounts of sucrose may pass into the intestine where they are broken down by other enzymes (sucrase or isomaltase glycoside hydrolases) located in the membrane of the microvilli lining the duodenum. These products are also transported rapidly into the bloodstream. Sucrose reaching the large intestine may also be digested by the enzyme invertase found in bacteria that reside there.

In human nutrition, sucrose is an easily assimilated macronutrient that provides a quick source of energy to the body, provoking a rapid rise in blood glucose upon ingestion. However, pure sucrose is not normally part of a human diet balanced for good nutrition, although it may be included sparingly to make certain foods more palatable.

Consider the following lengthy list of adverse effects of sugar (sucrose) from a March 1993 issue of the Townsend Letter for Doctors:

"Many of us have heard that if sugar were to attempt now to pass the FDA approval process it would not be approved. . . They (the FDA) give a list of ways in which sugar is known to be harmful. The reactions they list are: immune system suppression; mineral imbalance; hyperactivity; rise in triglycerides; reduces defenses against infection; reduces high density lipoproteins; chromium an copper deficiency; cancer of the breast, ovaries, intestines, prostate and rectum; increases fasting levels of glucose and insulin; interferes with absorption of calcium and magnesium; weakens eyesight; raises serotonin; causes hypoglycemia; produces stomach over-acidity; increases adrenalin levels; produces anxiety, irritability and difficulty concentrating; aging; alcoholism; tooth decay; obesity; contributes to duodenal and gastric ulcers; arthritis; asthma; Candida albicans (yeast infections); gallstones; heart disease; appendicitis; multiple sclerosis; hemorrhoids; varicose veins; elevates glucose and insulin responses in conjunction with the use of contraceptives; periodontal disease; osteoporosis; decrease in insulin sensitivity and glucose tolerance; decrease in growth hormone; increases cholesterol and systolic blood pressure; drowsiness and decreased activity; migraine headaches; food allergies; contributes to diabetes; toxemia during pregnancy; eczema, and it interferes with protein absorption." [43]

High sugar consumption is associated with the development of insulin resistance and contributes to development of the metabolic syndrome.[44] This condition or syndrome is approaching epidemic proportions in the United States.

"The insulin resistance syndrome (syndrome X or the metabolic syndrome) has become a major health problem of our times. Associated obesity, dyslipidemia, atherosclerosis, hypertension, and Type 2 Diabetes conspire to shorten life spans, while hyperandrogenism with polycystic ovarian syndrome affect the quality of life and fertility of increasing numbers of women."[45]

The rapidity with which sucrose raises blood glucose levels can cause problems for people suffering from defects in glucose metabolism. In an experiment with rats fed a diet one-third of which was sucrose, the sucrose first elevated levels of triglycerides in the blood. As triglycerides were transported into the cells, they induced formation of visceral fat and ultimately resulted in insulin resistance.[46] Such results were consistent with other studies that found that rats fed sucrose-rich diets developed high triglycerides, hyperglycemia, and insulin resistance.[47]

Sucrose, as a pure carbohydrate, has an energy content of nearly four Calories per gram (actually 3.94 kilocalories or 17 kilojoules per gram). When foods containing a high percentage of sucrose are consumed, many beneficial and required nutrients may be displaced from the diet, thus contributing to increased risks for several chronic diseases including diabetes, cardiovascular disease, some forms of cancers, osteoporosis and even chronic neuro-degenerative diseases.

High Fructose Corn Syrup (HFCS)

HFCS 55 (the HFCS most commonly used in foods and in food manufacturing) is 55% fructose and 45% glucose, again nearly a one-to-one ratio similar to that found in honey. When ingested, the glucose and fructose from HFCS pass through the stomach and are rapidly absorbed into the bloodstream from the small intestine, very similar to the glucose and fructose from honey or sucrose.

Beginning in the 1970s, HFCS became the sweetener of choice for most soft drink manufacturers. HFCS now represents greater than 40% of caloric sweeteners added to foods and drinks and is the sole caloric sweetener in soft drinks in the United States. In 2006, the daily per capita consumption of soft drinks was 17.8 ounces or nearly one and one half cans of pop per day per man, woman and child. *A conservative estimate of the consumption of HFCS indicates a daily average of 1320 calories for all Americans aged two years and above. The top 20% consumers of caloric sweeteners ingest a whopping 3160 calories from HFCS per day.*[48]

Another study published in July 2007 reported the following:

"Of the nearly 9000 middle-aged men and women who participated in the study, those who said they drank one pop or more per day had:

- A 31 per cent greater chance of developing obesity;
- A 30 per cent increased risk for gaining inches around the waist;
- A 25 per cent chance of developing high blood sugar levels
- A 32 per cent greater chance of developing lower "good" cholesterol (HDL) levels.

The one-or-more-a–day consumers were compared to non-frequent consumers, and adjustments were made for total caloric intake, saturated and trans-fat intake, dietary fiber consumption, physical activity and smoking.

'Our study was observational, and so right now all we demonstrate is an association. We have not proven causality,' said Dr. Ravi Dhingra, lead author of the study and an instructor in medicine at Harvard Medical School."[49]

We know from these observation and other clinical experiments that the metabolic results of ingesting these three substances, honey, sucrose or HFCS, each with similar glucose and fructose content, are not the same! There is something quite different going on with regards to insulin and blood sugar responses, fat metabolism, fat storage, and resultant obesity in both children and adults who consume large quantities of sucrose and HFCS. While little distinction can be made between honey, sucrose and HFCS when comparing the sugar content of each, the short term and long term effects within the human system of consuming them are significantly different.

Chi-Tang Ho and his colleagues at Rutger's University found that soft drinks sweetened with HFCS are up to ten times richer in harmful carbonyl compounds, such as methylglyoxal, than a diet soft drink control.[50] Carbonyl compounds are known to be elevated in individuals with diabetes and are blamed for causing diabetic complications such as foot ulcers and eye and nerve damage.[51, 52] Similar levels of carbonyl compounds are not found in table sugar but may be found in certain honey varietals.

The Problem with Fructose

To gain understanding of what may underlie the problems associated with sucrose and HFCS, we will take an isolated look at fructose and its observed effects on the human system.

Chronic excess fructose consumption has been suggested as the cause of insulin resistance (IR), obesity,[53, 54] elevated LDL cholesterol and triglycerides, and lead to other conditions associated with the metabolic syndrome. The fact that IR has risen in step with the increase in sugar and HFCS consumption cannot be disputed. However, the association, though strong, is not absolute. Short-term trials, lack of dietary controls, and lack of a non-fructose consuming control group are all confounding factors in human experiments. However, there are now a number of reports showing correlation of fructose consumption to obesity[55, 56, 57] especially central obesity, which is generally regarded as the most dangerous type. Other studies have linked the increased amounts of fructose from HFCS to changes in blood lipid profiles, among other things.

There is an additional concern with Type 1 diabetic patients and fructose. Physicians and nutritionists have recommended fructose as an alternative sweetener for diabetics due its Glycemic Index (GI) being significantly lower than glucose, sucrose and starches.

The problem here is that the GI is an incomplete and perhaps inappropriate standard of comparison. In calculating the GI, the body's blood glucose response is "standardized" with *50 grams of glucose*. Applied nutrition research typically uses *50 grams of digestible carbohydrate* as a reference quantity in comparing GI. The basic GI definition is thus inconsistent and does not fully take into consideration glycemic load, rates of absorption and metabolism and where fructose is concerned, little consideration is given to the unique and lengthy metabolic pathway of fructose which involves phosphorylation and a multi-step enzymatic process in the liver.

"The medical profession thinks fructose is better for diabetics than sugar," says Meira Field, PhD, a research chemist at the USDA, "but every cell in the body can metabolize glucose. However, all fructose must be metabolized in the liver. The liver of the rats on the high fructose diet looked like the livers of alcoholics, plugged with fat and cirrhotic." [58]

Though it is not entirely true that all fructose is metabolized in the liver (other tissues such as the cells of the intestine, and sperm cells do use fructose directly as the main energy source), a large fructose load presents the liver with a challenge. "When fructose reaches the liver," says Dr. William J. Whelan, a biochemist at the University Of Miami School Of Medicine, "the liver goes bananas and stops everything else to metabolize the fructose." [59]

Several studies have attempted to identify the physiologic reasons by which fructose differs from glucose. After a meal, fructose, as compared to glucose, seems to result in lower circulating insulin levels. Leptin and ghrelin levels - hormones responsible for the control of appetite and satiety - are also lower after fructose consumption.[60] Therefore, It is hypothesized that eating lots of fructose could increase the likelihood of weight gain.[61, 62] Another study from *The American Journal of Clinical Nutrition* indicates that, "fructose given alone increased the blood glucose almost as much as a similar amount of glucose (78% of the glucose-alone area)."[63]

Fructose is a reducing sugar, as are all monosaccharides. The spontaneous addition of single sugar molecules to proteins, known as glycation, is a significant cause of damage in diabetics. Fructose appears to be as dangerous as glucose in this regard, so it does not seem to be a better answer for diabetes for this reason alone.[64] This may be an important contribution to senescence and many age-related chronic diseases.[65]

A study in mice suggests that fructose increases obesity.[66] Another study concluded that fructose "produced significantly higher fasting plasma triacylglycerol values than did the glucose diet in men" and "if plasma triacylglycerols are a risk factor for cardiovascular disease, then diets high in fructose may be undesirable."[67] Bantle and associates "noted the same effects in a study of 14 healthy volunteers who sequentially ate a high-fructose diet and one almost devoid of the sugar."[68]

Studies that have compared HFCS (a primary ingredient in soft drinks sold in the US) to sucrose find that they have essentially identical physiological effects. For instance, Melanson et al (2006), studied the effects of HFCS and sucrose sweetened drinks on blood glucose, insulin, leptin, and ghrelin levels. They found no significant differences in any of these parameters.[69] This is not surprising since sucrose as we have stated above is a disaccharide that digests to 50% glucose and 50% fructose; while the high fructose corn syrup most commonly used on soft drinks is similar in composition with 55% fructose and 45% glucose.

Furthermore, fructose chelates minerals in the blood. This effect is especially important with micronutrients such as copper, chromium and zinc. Since these solutes are normally present in small quantities, chelation of small numbers of ions may lead to deficiency diseases, immune system impairment and even insulin resistance, a component and precursor of Type 2 Diabetes.[70]

Metabolic Differences between Honey, Sugar, and HFCS

It is one thing to observe and document the differences of honey, sucrose, and HFCS on measurable parameters within the human system. It is quite another to explain the mechanisms of action that are responsible for these differences. Though our knowledge here is incomplete, there are a few clues that may explain these apparently contradictory observations in human metabolism.

Transport and Absorption Rates

Transport and absorption rates may give us the first clue. In the stomach and the lumen of the duodenum and small intestine, the oligo- and poly-saccharides (complex sugars) are broken down to monosaccharides (glucose and fructose) by glycoside hydrolase and the pancreatic and intestinal glycosidases. Glucose and fructose have their own specific transport proteins (GLUT-2 and GLUT-4 for glucose and GLUT-5 for fructose[71]) that facilitate their movement across the cell wall lining the small intestine (enterocyte) membranes. *However fructose may also be transported by GLUT-2 for which it competes with glucose and galactose.* It may be that this existence of dual transport proteins gives fructose a slight edge in absorption rates.

Fructose also seems to be absorbed by a passive transport mechanism, that is, it passes through the gut wall by a concentration gradient from high in the gut to lower in the gut cell and then across the cell to the membrane of the blood vessels. If in fact, fructose is absorbed from the small intestine at higher concentrations and rates than glucose, this may provide a key as to why honey, sucrose and HFCS have differing effects on blood glucose levels and other metabolic parameters in the human.

Glycemic Load

If in fact fructose has an edge in absorption due to both active protein transport and passive diffusion due to concentration gradients, the amount of fructose presented to the circulation and then to the portal circulation would be quite different when one ingests a tablespoon of honey (about eighteen grams of carbohydrate of which only eight and a half grams is fructose) versus a liter of soft drink containing nearly 100 grams carbohydrate (50 grams of fructose) or a liter-and-a-half of soft drink containing nearly 150 grams of carbs (75 grams of fructose) - what in the U.S. is often referred to as the "Big Gulp ®."[72]

Could this massive amount of fructose that hits the circulation (nearly 10 times as much in the illustration above) after consuming a Big Gulp® be one key to why the liver rapidly metabolizes the fructose into trioses which result in elevated triglycerides while the smaller controlled amount of fructose from ingestion of a tablespoon of honey allows for the release of glucokinase from the hepatocyte nucleus that allows conversion of glucose to glycogen? We do know that the liver essentially stops everything else that it is doing when presented with a fructose load in order to metabolize it. Perhaps smaller amounts of fructose as presented by honey or a single serving of fruit do not present the liver with so great a challenge.

However, we cannot just talk about high fructose loads in isolation forgetting that with HFCS sweetened soft drinks and foods, there is also a massive amount of glucose ingested. This excessive amount of glucose triggers a huge insulin spike (actually an over production of insulin) which drives glucose immediately from the circulation into the cells where most of it is stored as fat. Meanwhile, the liver is trying to get rid of the high fructose load by breaking it into trioses (three carbon molecules) that enter directly into the formation of triglycerides. Thus we have a double whammy of fat formation from HFCS.

Following the ingestion of high sugar loads from sucrose or HFCS by about 90 minutes, the blood sugar level begins to drop due to the high insulin spike. By that time, however, the liver has not been able to replenish its glycogen stores (due to the excessive fructose load), and another event occurs. The liver is responsible for alerting the brain to the declining glycogen availability. It does this by releasing another protein called Insulin-like Growth Factor Binding Protein-1 or IGFBP-1. IGFBP-1 triggers the brain to begin preparing for a fuel shortage crisis. As IGFBP-1 is released from the liver, the brain responds by triggering the release of cortisol from the adrenal glands, which initiates the breakdown of the body's protein from muscle tissue to form glucose. This metabolic stress repeated day after day, year after year, may be what in fact is happening over time that contributes to the development of insulin resistance and subsequently to the onset of diabetes. Normally we do not ingest honey in the massive amounts that we do with sucrose or HFCS. However, matching GI and glycemic loads should produce similar effects, but they don't. Same sugars - different effects! Clearly the liver must be the key factor. Something happens to fructose derived from honey that is different from fructose derived from sucrose or HFCS when ingested in the same quantity. But what? And how is the difference explained?

We do know that something very big, very significant, is going on in the liver because fructose from either sucrose or HFCS is converted primarily to fat. Such is not the case with fructose from honey. There is something in honey that allows the liver metabolize fructose in the way nature intended that is not found in other refined or artificial sweeteners. Truly honey is an amazing, miraculous food.

We do not have all the answers at this point. There is still work that has to be done, but clearly there are metabolizing principles involved that improve glucose/fructose metabolism from honey in the liver in a way that glucose/ fructose from others sugars simply cannot match! Something in honey allows the liver to both form glycogen *and* prevent a rapid rise in blood glucose at the same time. Because liver glycogen is formed, and as a result no IGFBP-1 is released, the brain does not initiate the release of adrenal hormones, and as a result, insulin resistance does not develop.

It may be that there are combinations of mechanisms at work to explain the differences. In summary, these may include one or more of the following:

- Variances in transport / absorption rates
- Differences in Glycemic Index (GI) and Glycemic Load
- The rate of glycogen formation in liver
- Antioxidant content of honey and reduced oxidative stress in the tissues in general and
- The presence of other bioactive principles found in honey such as zinc, copper and their effect on B-cells in the pancreas

More study is necessary to refine the mechanisms that differentiate honey from sugar and HFCS. However, results from observational studies in both humans and animals can give us confidence now that honey is by far a superior food and should be preferred for regular consumption.

4 Unmasking the Pretenders

Chapter Summary

There are over twenty natural sugar substitutes and about ten artificial sweeteners that have been identified and produced in the past forty years. A few have had some share of the market for artificial sweeteners. Individuals with impairments in glucose tolerance or others who are simply being "calorie conscious" use these substitutes frequently without knowledge of their effects on the body.

Recent studies have begun to point out an alarming observation. Weight gain, rather than weight loss, is associated with the consumption of some sugar substitutes. Many of these products have significant glycemic load. Others result in a pronounced insulin effect in spite of the fact that they "contain no sugar" or do not raise blood sugar levels.

This chapter will unmask these pretenders and explain why honey should be the sweetener of choice for diabetics and those wanting to lose weight.

The headlines are eye catching:

> "New Sweetener Approved with No Calories, No Carbohydrates"

> "FDA-Approved Sweetener - Safe for Diabetics"

The tag lines are equally impressive:

> ". . .an all-natural sweetener that looks exactly like honey, tastes exactly like honey, and has the same consistency as honey. *In fact, it's putting bees out of business*."

"Made from sugar so it tastes like sugar."

Marketing is all about perception. It is no mistake that the marketing of various artificial sweeteners attempts to change perceptions, i.e. making something seem to be something that it is not.

Another way of making this point is to ask the question "When is a carbohydrate not a carbohydrate?" Answer: "When it is called by a different name and defined in different terms." The companies that manufacture artificial sweeteners have been at this for years, at least since the 1950s when such substances were first approved for human consumption.

In Chapter 2 we briefly discussed the basic fuels that the body uses for energy. There are only three - carbohydrates, proteins, and fats. The manufacturers of artificial sweeteners would have us to believe that they have invented a new food group, something that tastes like sugar, but has no carbohydrates and no calories, something that is made from sugar but is not sugar.

The problem is that half-truths are not entirely true! Half-truths are by definition half lies or at best distortions of truth intended to deceive the uninformed consumer.

There are several substances that have been used as artificial sweeteners over the past forty years. Some are naturally occurring substances or *natural* sugar substitutes. The list includes *sugar alcohols* like maltitol, lactitol, mannitol, sorbitol, glycerol and xylitol. All are in fact carbohydrates or derived from carbohydrates. Then there are several sweet plant *proteins* or *glycoproteins* (long chains of amino acids or amino acid-carbohydrate chains) like brazzein (1994), curculin (1990), monellin (1969), thaumatin (1990), mabinlin (1983), pentadin (1989) and miraculin (1989). Finally there are other soluble *dietary fibers* like polydextrose. Some on this list can be synthesized in a manufacturing process cheaper than they can be extracted from plants. For a list of natural sugar substitutes and a comparison of their sweetness by weight to sucrose, see Appendix B.

The process of determining the usefulness or healthfulness of these sugar substitutes, whether natural or artificial, should include an understanding of the effects on the body of these substances. This is critical as sugar substitutes have been in widespread use by individuals concerned about their weight since the 1970s. The use of these sugar substitutes has mushroomed within the "diet-food" industry. They have also been recommended by medical and health professionals for use with persons with glucose metabolism impairments and diabetes. But are they beneficial for weight loss?[73] Do they help lower blood sugar levels in diabetics? In order to answer these questions, the additional following questions should be answered for each of these substances:

- How are these substances absorbed into the circulation from the gut?

- Where in the gut does this absorption take place?

- What metabolites do they produce while in the gut, if any?

- What is the glycemic load (calorie load) from ingesting these substances?

- What is the insulin response (insulin index) from ingesting foods containing these substances?

Natural Sugar Substitutes

Sugar Alcohols

Sugar alcohol is a form of carbohydrate. Sugar alcohols as a group are generally not as sweet as sucrose. They are frequently used to mask the aftertastes of some artificial sweeteners as their flavor is like sucrose. One advantage of sugar alcohols is that they are not metabolized by the bacteria in the mouth and therefore do not cause tooth decay. Because of this they are used as sweeteners in chewing gum and hard candy.

The caloric impact of sugar alcohols is not zero as some food manufactures would have you believe. If that were true, the glycemic index (GI) would be zero. (Only two sugar alcohols have a GI of zero, according to research published by Geoffrey Livesey in 2003. These are mannitol and erythritol.[74]) But in fact, the GI of intermediate maltitol syrup, a commonly used sugar alcohol, is 53, which is higher than that of pasta, orange juice, or most vegetables. Maltitol syrup also provides three quarters of the energy value as an equivalent amount of sucrose (3 Calories per gram versus 4).

Because sugar alcohols are not completely absorbed into the blood stream from the small intestines, they reach the large intestine where bacterial action can lead to bloating, diarrhea and flatulence. Metabolites of sugar alcohols also enter the fatty acid metabolic chain forming triglycerides and can contribute to elevated fatty acid levels in the blood and increased fat storage.

One product that utilizes sugar alcohol as a sweetener is something that is sold as "sugar-free honey." You can buy it in the big box stores. It is inexpensive. The manufacturer will tell you that the product is safe for diabetics because it contains no sugar. Brilliant marketing! The truth is that the product is not honey and contains no honey! While it is technically true that it contains no sugar or sucrose, the truth is distorted by redefining the word sugar.

The product gets its sweetness from a sugar alcohol, maltitol. Maltitol is just as much a sugar as it is a carbohydrate. Maltitol is a disaccharide (literally two sugars) made by hydrogenation of maltose obtained from starch, a carbohydrate. Multiple published articles indicate that maltitol and its syrups do have a considerable effect on blood glucose levels.[75, 76] And some maltitol is metabolized in the large intestine, a process that produces triglycerides that contribute to the formation of fats. Neither elevation of blood sugar levels nor additional fat formation should be considered healthful or safe for diabetics.

Glycerin

Glycerin (or glycerol) is also a sugar alcohol used as a sugar substitute. It actually has more calories (27) per teaspoon than table sugar even though it is only 60% as sweet as sucrose. However, it does not raise blood sugar levels, nor does it feed the bacteria that form plaques and cause dental cavities. In addition to its use as a sweetener, glycerin is used as a solvent, antifreeze, plasticizer, drug medium, and in the manufacture of soaps, cosmetics, inks, lubricants, and dynamite.

Dr. Thomas Wolever, professor and acting chair of the department of nutritional sciences at the University of Toronto, indicated in a published article in 2005 that glycerin did not have a significant effect on blood sugar levels nor did it prompt an insulin response.[77] It does however have an effect on the liver. Like fructose, the liver is the only place in the body that can metabolize glycerol. Glycerol is a precursor for synthesis of triacylglycerols and of phospholipids in the liver and adipose tissue.

Polydextrose

Polydextrose is another carbohydrate used as a sugar substitute. As a food ingredient it is classified as a soluble fiber and is frequently used to increase the fiber content of food, reduce calories and reduce fat content. It is synthesized from dextrose (glucose) to which is added about ten percent sorbitol and one percent citric acid. The energy value of polydextrose is only one Calorie per gram, about one-fourth the caloric value of sucrose. The FDA approved it as a food ingredient in 1981.

In some animal studies, polydextrose has been found to cause changes to the morphology of the large intestine, suggesting that polydextrose should be used carefully as a dietary fiber-like substance in food manufacturing.[78]

Polydextrose is not absorbed directly into the circulation from the intestine. It does contribute to the glycemic load, but only at one-fourth the calories of sucrose. There may also be an insulin response associated with the ingestion of polydextrose.

Stevia

Stevia is not approved as a sugar substitute in the United States, but it is available as a food supplement. The distinction may be subtle and confusing but the fact remains that in the United States, it is legal to import, grow, sell, and consume products containing stevia which are labeled for use as a dietary supplement, but not as a food additive. It is banned for use in food in the European Union, Singapore and Hong Kong. It has been approved as a dietary supplement in Australia, New Zealand and Canada. In Japan and South American countries, stevia may also be used as a food additive.

What exactly is this sweet plant food substance that causes such controversy around the world? Stevia comes from a group of plant species of herbs or shrubs in the sunflower family (Asteraceae), native to subtropical and tropical South America and Central America. It is widely cultivated and used for food in parts of Asia including China, Malaysia, and Thailand. One species of Stevia, commonly known as sweet leaf, sugarleaf, or simply stevia, is specifically grown for its sweet leaves. Stevia is about 300 times sweeter than sucrose though some of its extracts may have a bitter or licorice-like aftertaste at high concentrations. Stevia is widely used as a sweetener in Japan.

Rebiana is the trade name for a patent-pending, calorie-free, food and beverage sweetener derived from stevia and developed jointly by The Coca-Cola Company and Cargill. In May 2007, Coca-Cola™ announced plans to obtain approval for its use as a food additive within the United States by 2009.[79] Coca-Cola™ has also announced plans to market rebiana-sweetened products in 12 countries that allow stevia's use as a food additive. The two companies are conducting their own studies in an effort to gain regulatory approval in the United States and the European Union.[80]

Stevia has a negligible effect on blood glucose, even enhancing glucose tolerance.[81] Once given more widespread approval, it could be more attractive as a natural sweetener and therefore gain approval for diabetics and others on carbohydrate-controlled diets.[82]

Artificial Sugar Substitutes

Saccharin

Saccharin[83] is the oldest known artificial sweetener, produced first in 1878. Its use did not become widespread until sugar shortages during the period of World War I. Since the 1950s, Saccharin or benzoic sulfinide as it is known chemically, has been produced synthetically. During the 1960s, its popularity increased among dieters as a calorie-free sweetener. It is about 300 times as sweet as sucrose, yet has effectively no food energy, that is, it passes through the human digestive system undigested. Because of its unpleasant aftertaste, it is frequently combined with other artificial sweeteners such as aspartame or cyclamate in countries where these are permitted as food additives.

Although saccharin ingestion results in no metabolites or provides no caloric load, it does trigger an insulin response. [See Gustatory Insulin Effect below.]

Aspartame

Aspartame was first discovered in 1965 and first given approval for use as an artificial sweetener in dry food products in 1981. It was approved for use in carbonated beverages in 1983. The FDA reemoved all restrictions for its use in 1996 making it available for use in all foods. The U.S. patent for aspartame expired in 1992. A number of companies currently market the product under a number of brand or trademark names including Tropicana Slim, Equal, NutraSweet, and Canderel. It is used as a sweetener in approximately 6,000 consumer foods and beverages sold worldwide.

Aspartame has a caloric value of 4 kilocalories (17 kilojoules) per gram, exactly the same as sucrose, however the quantity of aspartame needed to produce a sweet taste is so small that in typical use its caloric contribution is negligible. Aspartame is roughly 180 times as sweet as sugar in usual concentrations which makes it a popular sweetener for those trying to avoid calories. It is also used by diabetics as a sugar substitute. In spite of its low calorie content, aspartame does trigger an insulin effect which is described below.

Sucralose

Sucralose (or Splenda as it was called under its original trademark) was approved for use in the United States in 1998. It is approximately 600 times as sweet as sugar. Even though sucralose is made from sugar, it should not be considered a natural product. It is manufactured by selectively adding chlorine atoms to sucrose, replacing the hydroxyl groups. Though sucralose contains 86% of the calories of sugar, it is only about 15% as dense meaning that a given volume only has about 12% the caloric energy as the same volume of sugar. Sucralose actually contains 1.66 Calories per teaspoon compared to about 18 Calories per teaspoon for sugar. The small individual-sized packets of Splenda contain 3.31 Calories but under the FDA's labeling regulations, the calorie content is listed as "zero calories."[84]

Because of its super-sweetness, Splenda as sold in those small tear-open packets contains a relatively small amount of sucralose. The calories come from the highly fluffed filler or carrier (dextrose or maltodextrin) with which the sucralose is mixed to give it its volume. Dextrose and maltodextrin each have 3.75 calories per gram. When ingested, only about 20% of sucralose is absorbed and only 20 to 30% of that is metabolized[85] thus making sucralose a suitable replacement for calorie conscious individuals. As with other artificial sweeteners, ingestion of sucralose does trigger an insulin effect.

The Gustatory Insulin Effect

In recent years, investigators have discovered that insulin is released from the pancreas gland in response to taste. In other words, insulin release occurs independently of rising blood glucose levels. Several studies have documented the fact that insulin is released simply from the stimulation of sweetness receptors on the tongue.[86, 87] This is a significant fact regarding most artificial sweeteners, one that is not yet widely appreciated. We call this the *gustatory insulin effect*.

At least two different sweetness receptors found primarily on the tongue need to be activated for the brain to register sweetness. While this fact may seem insignificant to the average dieter indulging in supposedly calorie-free or low calorie diet foods and drinks, it becomes quite relevant because of its impact on circulating blood sugar levels.

Several artificial sweeteners in widespread use in the United States and Canada have the ability to activate these sweetness receptors and thus trigger a release of insulin. These include saccharin, cyclamate (Sweet'N Low® in Canada[88]), aspartame (Equal or NutraSweet), acesulfame potassium (Sunett, Sweet One), sucralose (Splenda), and neotame (NutraSweet).

To illustrate, suppose one consumes a diet drink without any additional caloric input. Though there are no readily available nutrients (carbohydrates or sugars) that would typically trigger an immediate insulin response to rising blood glucose levels, insulin *is* released as a result of the activation of sweetness receptors on the tongue. Even though no actual calories have been ingested, circulating glucose (which remains in the blood stream at levels between 80 and 110 mg/dl) is now being driven into the cells by the insulin released as a result of consuming this diet drink.

Insulin's function is always the same – drive glucose into the cells where it can be used for energy. If the body is at rest, glucose may not be needed immediately (typically there is more circulating glucose than is needed for energy requirements) and the excess glucose is then converted to glycogen in the muscle cells and/or stored as fat for later use. In effect, insulin is a fat storing hormone.

In the case of beverages or foods containing these artificial sweeteners, the insulin release prompted by the sweetness receptors on the tongue stimulates fat storage even when few or no calories are being ingested!

Metabolic Hazards of Diet Drinks

Stating this another way, diet drinks (and foods containing artificial sweeteners for that matter), in spite of their lower calorie status, may play a significant role in causing fat formation and storage by way of their gustatory insulinic effect. In fact, similar metabolic hazards (increased prevalence of the metabolic syndrome,[89] higher risk of obesity, [90, 91] high blood pressure,[92] and diabetes mellitus[93]) are more common in individuals consuming soft drinks. It seems to make little difference in the associated risk, incidence or prevalence of these conditions whether the drink is regular or diet among those who have at least one-and-a-half cans of these beverages per day. The only logical conclusion one can draw from this similarity is that sweetness receptors, without regard to type of sweetener ingested, trigger an insulin response which drives glucose into the cells where it is stored as fat.

As we indicated in Chapter 3, many studies have shown the association between obesity and consumption of diet drinks. Many diabetic patients who have been instructed by their doctors or dietitians to use artificial sweeteners have been perplexed by their inability to lose weight. Most continue to gain weight primarily because they follow the very advice aimed at reducing caloric input.[94]

Given the fact that some artificial sweeteners are metabolized directly to triglycerides and others stimulate insulin release, it is not surprising that diabetic patients and dieters using these products continue to have elevated serum triglycerides, store more fat, and continue to gain weight.

5 Fueling for Health Begins at Bedtime

Chapter Summary

The fact that duration and quality of sleep are factors contributing to optimum health is not surprising. Sleep is an energy-driven process requiring proper fuel during the night fast. Recent research points to short or poor quality sleep as a risk factor for diabetes, obesity, hypertension, cardiovascular disease and other metabolic conditions.

Restorative sleep is critical for memory, cognitive enhancement and offline processing as well as all of the reparative functions necessary for muscle, bone and other tissues. Mechanisms triggered by light/dark cycles mediated by nuclei in the brain allow this to happen when the brain is provided with optimum fuel from adequate liver glycogen stores during rest.

Consuming honey before bedtime helps initiate and sustain restorative sleep and insures other health benefits while preventing the cumulative ravages of metabolic stress during the night fast.

Sleep, although taking up around one third of our lives, remains one of the least charted and least understood aspects of human physiology, in spite of several decades of sleep research. Several aspects of sleep and sleep physiology require further research and investigation. This chapter concerns itself with some of these critical aspects of sleep, including its:

- restorative functions,
- role in information processing, dreams, memory consolidation and retrieval,
- metabolic environment, fuel requirements and energy homeostasis, and
- role in immune system modulation.

Professor William Dement, the grandfather of sleep research, noted as far back as the 1970s that patients sent to him suffering from narcolepsy were usually suffering from sleep apnea. It was also observed that most of these patients were overweight. These observations were the first clue that sleep was somehow related to weight and appetite control. His findings also led others to investigate the impact of poor quality sleep on energy homeostasis and metabolic conditions. Sleep discovery research conducted during the last few years has resulted in major steps forward linking short and poor quality sleep to various metabolic syndromes.

The Critical Role of Liver Glycogen

The critical role of liver glycogen as the primary fuel for the brain was introduced in Chapter 2. Here we underscore this important physiologic principle as it relates to the period of the night fast. The adult liver releases approximately ten grams of glycogen or glucose each hour, two-thirds of which is needed to provide the brain with a stable energy supply during the eight hours of sleep. The other third is used to provide energy to the kidneys and red blood cells. This liver glycogen store also plays a crucial role in stabilizing the blood glucose concentration during rest. The liver can store between 75 and 100 grams of glycogen or about eight percent of its total weight after a meal. But remember that it gives up ten grams per hour to supply the energy needs of the brain, kidneys and red blood cells.

In view of the modern propensity not to eat late in the evening, a habit resulting from our belief in the myth that food eaten before bed will turn to fat, most of our western populations retire to bed with a partially depleted liver glycogen store. And as a result, metabolic stress is increased during the late night or early morning hours. Recovery physiology, which should take place during rest, is impeded. Many suffer from poor quality sleep and/or short sleep experiencing increased risk for a series of adrenal driven diseases characterized as the metabolic syndrome (see End Note 1 for a detailed description of the metabolic syndrome). The best known of these conditions is obesity, Type 2 Diabetes, hypertension and heart disease.

When We Go to Sleep the Body Goes to Work

Sleep is an energy-driven physiological process. When we retire to bed, our body goes (or should go) to work! This simple statement of scientific fact contradicts much of modern popular thinking regarding what exactly happens during the eight hours of the night fast. This thinking is based on the notion that because no physical exercise occurs, sleep is a process that somehow uses little or no energy. From this we wrongly conclude that eating in the period prior to bed will result in food being converted into fat and stored in the adipose tissue. This is usually expressed in the myth referenced above that "food eaten late in the evening will just turn to fat." Nothing could be further from the scientific truth. Food is digested and absorbed at night in exactly the same way as it is during the daytime, perhaps even better because the circadian rythm controling adrenal hormone release ensures reduction of these hormones during that time.

But there is one caveat to this situation. Much of the energy required during sleep for the brain, kidneys and red blood cells must be sourced from the liver. Quality, healthful, restorative sleep is dependent on adequate stock of liver glycogen. To avoid triggering metabolic stress, the liver glycogen store must be "topped off" prior to bed. Restorative sleep fueled by adequate liver glycogen during the period of the night fast promotes recovery physiology. Recovery physiology is repairative - a vigorous rebuilding and restorative activity affecting all tissues in the body.

Recovery physiology is primarily fat-burning physiology utilizing fat stores for energy requirements. But fat-burning physiology functions at rest only when the brain is provided with adequate glycogen supply to get through the night. By consciously restocking the liver prior to bedtime with *honey* - the ideal liver/brain food - we activate the Honey/Insulin/Melatonin (HYMN) Cycle [See Appendix E, Poster No 14]. This wonderful metabolic cycle promotes quality, healthful, restorative sleep. Restorative sleep prompts recovery and fat-burning physiology.

Sleep and the Metabolic Syndrome – The Connections

There is little question that the quality of one's sleep is profoundly related to the widespread prevalence of certain metabolic conditons in our population, notably obesity and diabetes. In a presentation given to the 10th European Congress of Endocrinology in May of 2008, Eve Van Cauter of the University of Chicago stated the following:

"Sleep curtailment has become a common behavior in industrialized countries. Simultaneously, the aging of the population is associated with an increased prevalence of sleep disturbances. These trends for shorter sleep duration and poorer sleep quality have developed over the same time period as the dramatic increase in the prevalence of obesity and diabetes. *There is recent evidence to indicate that chronic partial sleep loss and decreased sleep quality may increase the risk of obesity and diabetes* (emphasis added) . . . the current evidence suggests that chronic partial sleep curtailment, a novel behavior that appears to have developed with the advent of the 24-h society, and reduced sleep quality may be involved in the current epidemic of obesity and diabetes."[95] [The quote is reproduced in its entirety following the End Note.]

Sleep, Energy Status, and the Metabolic Syndrome - Connecting More Dots

The notion that sleep is an energy-driven process, in other words quality sleep is associated with a high energy status, is a notion that will confuse many of our modern dietary gurus. However, a growing body of science points to exactly this conclusion. This energy status is furthermore correlated with the glycogen plenitude in the liver. This profound connection seems to have been missed by the medical and scientific establishment for several decades.

Many studies, including those referenced by Professor Van Cauter in her presentation cited above, point to the connection between poor quality or shortened sleep and a cascade of modern metabolic disorders we refer to as the metabolic syndrome or syndrome X, including obesity, Type 2 Diabetes, and cardiovascular disease. [A more complete description of the metabolic syndrome is included in End Note 1.] However, the association that clearly links the "multiple factors that mediate this adverse impact of sleep loss" with metabolic stress ("increased sympathetic nervous activity, decreased brain glucose uptake and elevated evening cortisol levels") is stated without describing an underlying mechanism.

It is the liver glycogen store - the regulating factor for the body's energy status - that connects all of this together. The fact that the medical and scientific establishment have missed this connection most certainly can be traced to the lack of scientific interest in liver glycogen and its role in the physiology of sleep. Only in recent years have the metabolic dots begun to be gradually connected together.

In 1999, Professor Van Cauter and her team at Chicago University found that in otherwise healthy young men, a loss of four hours sleep each night for only six nights resulted in alteration of their metabolic profile from that of a healthful state to that consistant with obesity and Type 2 Diabetes.[96] This is an astonishing reversal of health over such a short period of time, and points out the devastating consequences of this form of metabolism experienced by many over months, years and even decades. Though this study did not point out an underlying mechanism for the observed disruption in the subject's metabolic profiles, it can be safely deduced that short sleep results in an increase of metabolic stress including increased sympathetic nervous system activity, disruptions in brain glucose uptake, and increased levels of circulating cortisol.

In January 2005, two physicians, Joseph Bass, MD and Fred W. Turek, MD published a seminal review entitled "Sleepless in America: a pathway to obesity and the metabolic syndrome?" In this wonderful paper they draw the connection between short and poor quality sleep, obesity and the metabolic syndrome. They state that according the National Sleep Foundation of America, children of all ages are sleeping one to two hours less per night than they require.

".... these remarkable, and at the same time surprising findings, led basic and clinical researchers off on the trail to find the physiological linkages between insufficient sleep and metabolic function. This work also renewed interest in the role of many of the metabolic abnormalities associated with sleep apnea. *However while there is growing awareness among some sleep, metabolic, cardiovascular and diabetes researchers that insufficient sleep could be leading to a cascade of disorders, few in the general medical profession or in the lay public have yet made the connection* (emphasis added)."[97]

Given the fact that the metabolic profile caused by short sleep time is similar to that caused by poor quality sleep and/or stressful sleep, the links can now be more firmly established. Modern metabolic malfunction and the diseases that accompany it are associated with both short and/or poor quality sleep. Furthermore, *the connection between inadequate liver glycogen stores and stressed overnight physiology completes the explanation and gives us a model linking the metabolic syndrome and shortened, disordered, or poor quality sleep.*

In the following sections, these links will be discussed in more detail. Specifically, we will explain why selectively refueling the liver with honey prior to bed improves the overnight physiological profile and reduces the risk of all the conditions associated with metabolic stress.

Sleep - the Long and the Short of It

The medical research literature contains a growing number of studies that demonstrate the direct association between poor quality and/or short sleep and a number of conditions included in the metabolic syndrome, such as obesity, Type 2 Diabetes, hypertension, and increased risk of heart disease. However there is also growing recognition of a link between these syndromes and *prolonged* sleep, or sleep lasting more than eight hours. In research presented to the British Sleep Society in September 2007, Professor Francesco Cappuccio of Warwick University stated:

"Short sleep has been shown to be a risk factor for weight gain, hypertension and Type 2 Diabetes sometimes leading to mortality but in contrast to the short sleep-mortality association it appears that no potential mechanisms by which long sleep could be associated with increased mortality have yet been investigated. Some candidate causes for this include depression, low socioeconomic status and cancer-related fatigue."[98]

The putative mechanism for the fact that long sleep periods also promote increased metabolic stress is essentially the same as that relating short sleep to metabolic stress. Both are actually a potent confirmation of the endocrine and glucocorticoid responses to deminishing liver glycogen stores. In the case of prolonged sleep, the response may in some cases be increased. As sleep is extended, epinephrine and cortisol release continues as the brain directs its quest for glucose producing increased metabolic stress.

The apparent contradictory opposition of these physiological processes, although intuitive, is illusory. Both short or poor quality sleep and prolonged sleep produce similar metabolic responses as the brain seeks to insure adequate glycogen stores to fuel its basic energy demands. The impact on morbidity and mortality seems to be the same from both sleep extremes. This observation provides clues to the mechanisms by which sleep disorders are associated with hypertension, cardiovascular disease, obestiy and diabetes.

Sleep and the Fatuous Fast

The modern prohibition about "not eating late" has in effect resulted in what is essentially a 12-hour fast as opposed to lesser periods of overnight fasting in premodern times. This fast typically begins in the evening following an early supper and lasts until breakfast in the morning. If breakfast is skipped as is often the case, it may go on even longer than 12 hours or more. Rather than resulting in weight loss, this fatuous fast activates stress physiology which in turn results in *increased level of stress hormones being released which drive up appetite, prompt food-seeking behavior and promote increased weight gain.*

The Liver Glycogen Link Restated

As suggested above most of our western populations retire to bed with a partially depleted liver glycogen store due to belief in the myth that eating late promotes fat storage. Then after only a few hours, a low liver glycogen status stimulates an adrenal response which releases endocrine and glucocorticoid hormones (one of the basic principles described in **The Hibernation Diet**). This situation then begs the question, how much greater will be the adrenal response when an individual sleeps for more than eight hours? Now we have a set of conditions which serve to superimpose chronic overnight metabolic stress on the normal circadian activation of adrenal hormone release early in the morning. In other words, an extended fast of more than eight hours results in even greater adrenal activation as the body works to maintain fuel homeostasis.

The direct link between inadequate liver glycogen plenitude and resulting metabolic stress confirms the central role of liver glycogen in preventing the conditions brought about by both short sleep and long sleep. Rather than being confounding, these seemingly contradictory extremes (short and long sleep) are unified by this observation regarding liver glycogen stores. Pre-bedtime fueling of the liver (preferably with honey) to insure adequate liver glycogen supply is crucial in the prevention of the conditions associated with metabolic stress.

At Close of Day

A consolidated period of sleep lasting eight hours is a relatively modern phenomenon, becoming more and more prevalent with the development of artificial lighting first from gas lamps and later with the advent of electricity. In pre-modern times our ancestors would retire as daylight waned and rise with the morning light. This social and cultural habit was associated with a very important physiological consideration. In those times the human circadian cycle was coupled with and regulated by the light-dark cycle, much more so than it is today.

Our ancestors would have experienced periods of segmented or divided sleep punctuated by a period of wakefulness. These two periods of sleep, known as "first sleep" and "second sleep" were well established in medieval England. They were also widely practiced and referred to in other European countries. The period between the two sleeps was known and appreciated as one of quiet reflection, relaxed semi-wakefulness, and included a time for eating.

This breaking of the night fast may be significant because the term we now use for the first meal of the day - "break fast" - may in fact relate to the earlier phase of wakefulness between the two periods of sleep. Early researchers into the history of sleep such a Roger E Ekirch,[99] suggested that food was taken during the interval between the first and second sleep. If so, this would have profound implications for our ancester's overnight physiology during which natural diurnal cycles were linked closely to times for eating.

The implication from this observation may be that an eight-plus hour fast is physiologically unnatural, especially in contemporary western society where we typically do not eat late in the evening. Our historical and natural physiology appears to be in conflict with this modern and wholly unscientific inclination. As a direct result of our modern calorie fetishism we are encouraged not to take carbohydrates from around 7:00 PM in the evening until we arise the following morning, a fast approaching 12 hours.

The only carbohydrate store in the human body able to release glucose to other organs and tissues during this period is the liver. Thus, as pointed out in many different sections of this book, the liver glycogen store capacity is the critical factor during any period of fasting insofar as the brain must rely on liver glycogen to maintain a continuous supply of glucose for fuel. This perspective is in line with the archeological and paleontological record, and in part explains just why our hunter-gatherer ancestors were healthier than their farming descendents.[100]

Siesta and the Heart

The word siesta is derived from the Latin "*hora sexta*" meaning sixth hour. Although most popularly associated with Spain, this mid-day nap typically lasting around 30 minutes, is a common practice across the Mediterranean culture, North Africa, the Middle East, Latin America and in several Asian cultures. Humans possess a powerful drive for sleep. This is counterbalanced by an equally strong drive for wakefulness. Both are experienced in cyclical variations during the 24 hours of the day. Many people experience a mild drop in blood glucose shortly after the midday meal which promotes a period of relaxation coinciding with siesta time.

A 2007 study from Greece led by Professor Dimitros Trichopoulos of Harvard and Athens medical schools demonstrated that a 30 minute siesta three times weekly significantly reduced the risk of heart attack particularly in working young men.[101] This was a large prospective study involving a total of 23,681 residents of Greece with no history of heart disease, stroke or cancer at enrollment. They were followed for 6.3 years. The researchers found that those who took naps of any frequency and duration had a 34% lower risk of dying from heart disease than those who did not. Those who took naps of more than 30 minutes three or more times weekly had a 37% lower risk. Among working men who took midday naps, there was a whopping 64% reduced risk of death with a 36% reduced risk among non-working men.

The authors make no connection between such a postprandial nap and any reduction in metabolic stress, as opposed to lifestyle stress. However a restocked liver glycogen store would provide exactly the correct metabolic profile for a short beneficial sleep. It is interesting to speculate as to whether a siesta prior to or after the midday meal would have had a different outcome, given controls for liver glycogen status. Clearly the metabolic profile at this time of day may have impact on the value of such a siesta. In any case, this study suggests that a midday siesta reduces risk of heart disease and mortality related to heart attaks.

The 24 Hour Society

A growing and potentially toxic social development in Western culture is the extension of time increasingly anchored to technological activity, whether related to work or recreation. Much research has been carried out into this round-the-clock "shift work" and its metabolic impact on health and safety. Shift work can cause the normal circadian rhythms (the internal 'body clock' governing processes) to conflict with one's daily schedule resulting in adverse health and safety issues. Shift work, and other wake/sleep time mismatches such as those caused by jet-lag or sleep deprivation are linked to a range of adverse health effects.

A report to the UK Parliamentary Office of Science and Technology, raised this alarm in pointing out the following physiological impacts of shift work and its increased health risks:

- A 40% increase in cardiovascular disease. Meals taken during the 'biological night' may contribute towards increased risk of heart disease.
- Reproductive problems: spontaneous abortion, low birth weight, retarded fetal development, prematurity and significantly increased risks of miscarriage. Studies of women working irregular or rotating shifts show increased incidence of severe menstrual pains.
- Evidence that shiftwork increases the risk of breast and colorectal cancer. The extent of this and its underlying mechanisms are not fully understood.
- Sleep loss and disruption (particularly with night shifts). A vicious cycle can develop where caffeine is needed for alertness during the day and alcohol or sleeping pills are used at night. Poor sleep is also related to higher rates of substance abuse.
- Gastrointestinal disorders. After sleep problems, these are the most frequently reported symptoms. Some studies have shown that 20–75% of shift workers with night work complain of appetite disturbance and gastrointestinal problems, compared with 10–25% of day, and shift workers without night work. Peptic ulcers are two to eight times more frequent amongst night shift workers.[102]

This report presents an alarming rise in poor health and safety that impacts mortality and feeds directly into the range of metabolic disorders characterized as the metabolic syndrome.

All of the factors that extend the waking hours, whether social, cultural, lifestyle, or work related, activate adrenal stress physiology and lead to foreshortened and poor quality sleep. Together these factors are driving humanity in a downward spiral of physiological and psychoneural malfunctioning resulting in worsening human mortality rates after several centuries of almost continuous improvement.

The Suprachiasmatic Nucleus (SCN) and the Hypocretins

Rather than describing miniature aliens from outer space and their mechanisms of space travel, these fifty cent words are actually inextricably related to sleep physiology, our internal clock, and energy metabolism. The SCN is a vital region of the brain located in the hypothalamus. It regulates the human circadian clock mechanism. To put it another way, the hormonal and neuronal activities generated in the SCN control many different body functions during a 24-hour light-dark cycle[103] including modulation of body temperature and production and release of cortisol and melatonin. The discovery of these SCN hormones (see text box on following page) in recent years has opened up a new field of study tracing the links between low energy status and locomotion/wakeful activity, and high energy status and sleep. These links have turned out to be precisely the opposite of popular modern thinking which have associated elevated energy status with exercise and low energy status with sleep.

The Suprachiasmatic Nucleus (SCN) and the Hypocretins

The SCN receives nerve inputs from the human retina by way of the optic nerve. This visual signaling pathway regulates the human CLOCK (circadian locomotor output cycles kaput) genes via a unique interlocking feedback loop[104] involving two other proteins known as PER (Period) and TIM (Timeless). These proteins regulate their own expression and dissolution over the 24 hour cycle moving from the cell cytoplasm into the SCN at night and out again during daylight.

The SCN also connects to a group of neurons in the lateral hypothalamus that secrete hormones known as hypocretins or orexins. These are appetite stimulating hormones which also stimulate wakefulness and energy expenditure.[105, 106] The hypocretins are in turn inhibited or made active respectively by leptin and ghrelin. Leptin is a hormone produced by fat cells and serves as a long-term internal measure of energy state. Gherlin is a short-term hormonal factor secreted by the stomach just before an expected meal and strongly stimulates appetite. The hypocretins are also activated by hypoglycemia (low blood sugar) and inhibited by the presence of glucose. Together these hormones and their continually oscillating feedback cycles represent a very important link between metabolism and sleep regulation.

The hypocretin/orexin neurons interact with various other brain nuclei that have important roles in wakefulness. These include the "dopamine, norepinephrine, histamine and acetylcholine systems which are essential in stabilizing wakefulness and sleep. Recent studies indicate that the hypocretins have a major role in integrating metabolic, circadian and sleep debt influences"[107] which determine one's awake, sleep or activity status.

This rather technical diversion into the complicated realm of brain function underscores a rather profound connection among wake/sleep states, appetite, glucose metabolism and modern metabolic malfunction.

Another Clue from Narcolepsy

One additional clue illustrating the inter-connectedness of appetite and sleep paterns comes from recent research that connects the hypocretins (hormones produced in the hypothalamus) to narcolepsy. Narcolepsy is a neurological condition in which one may fall asleep often at inappropriate times and places. This excessive daytime sleepiness (EDS) is coupled with nocturnal sleep disturbances, insomnia, and disrupted cycles of non-rapid eye movement (NREM) and rapid eye movement (REM) sleep. Narcoleptics have been shown to be deficient in the neurons in the brain which produce hypocretins, the neuropeptides responsible for wakefulness, energy expenditure and appetite.

This connection between narcolepsy, hypocretins, energy expenditure, appetite and locomotion opens a window into a deep, dynamic and seemingly contradictory physiological polarity. In narcolepsy we have a physiologic mechanism unable to function properly. This mechanism involves the hypocretins which as has been stated are associated with wakeful activity and food seeking. The result of this malfunction is that narcoleptics have a powerful and uncontrolable stimulous for sleep. The frustration of one element in this dynamic (energy expenditure and locomotion) appears to promote the opposite element (sleep). Perhaps even more surprising is that this obverse physiological dualism is modulated in the same region of the brain, the SCN.

Dr. Theodore B. VanItallie from St. Luke's-Roosevelt Hospital Center in New York refers to this physiologic dualism in a paper published in 2006:

"Early humans, in order to survive, needed to obtain food - most often by some form of hunting and/or gathering. Many of the sources of food sufficient to meet their energy needs must have required considerable physical exertion. To remain in energy equilibrium, the hunters/gatherers needed food in quantities sufficient to offset resting metabolic requirement, 'everyday' physical activity, and the extra energy cost of the physical activity imposed by food seeking. The amount and duration of exertion that the human body can endure without becoming severely fatigued is strictly limited; therefore, industrious food seekers had to rest periodically to permit restoration of their capacity for physical work."[108]

This connection, between locomotion/food seeking activity, appetite and sleep physiology as found in narcolepsy, provides yet another confirmation of the interrelatedness of our most profound physiological drives. It is essential that a restoration of energy homeostasis occur between our innate drives for activity and rest. That this unity and conflict of oppositional drives is mediated within the same physiologic entity, the SCN, is another marvel of creation.

Fueling the Control Center: The Missing Link - Liver Glycogen

The above discussion has primarily focused on the dynamic regulatory center which monitors and controls wake/sleep states, appeite, and energy expenditure. Now it is timely to revisit the energy store most critical to this physiologic dynamic. A control room without power is simply a room full of idle inert gagets. The incredible design of our human system includes an energy supply and status indicator that insures that the "control room" (the human brain) never runs out of power. This energy supply resides in the liver glycogen store. The store comes complete with an automatic energy staus indicator that warns of deminishing supplies.

The history of scientific interest in this fuel store begins in the 19th century with its discovery by Claude Barnard.[109] Following in the 1930s and 1940s were studies relating to the size and concentration of this energy storehouse. Then followed a period of relative scientific neglect that lasted for nearly fifty years with only some minor interest during the 1960s. The late 1990s and continuing into the early years of the 21st century witnessed renewed interest which has continued through the present. [See Historical Summary of Liver Glycogen - Energy Status Research in the text box which follows on page 59.]

Science, similar to other fields of human endeavor is subject to periods of fashion, periods of neglect, and periods of renewed interest. These cycles seemingly osscilate over many decades. However, the relative disinterest in the liver as a critical fuel supply depot may seem surprising in that its most important physiological role is to provide a continuous supply of glucose to the brain over the 24-hour cycle. Furthermore, the liver is the only glycogen store that can release glucose to other organs and tissues. The much larger glycogen store in muscle tissue remains in muscle cells and is not shared with other organs. Perhaps it is the fact that the liver is an organ with a wide range of physiological roles which include digestion, detoxification, bile formation, protein and fat synthesis, along with glycogen storage. These other activities may have, to some extent, obscured the importance of its role in glucose storage and metabolism. The one exception to this is the role of the liver in diabetes.

Not only does liver glycogen store play an essential role in the fueling the central control region of the brain (the SCN), it also is critical to recovery physiology and for providing energy for what we refer to as metabolic or physiologic stress. Though psychologic stress may be significant and profoundly interlinked with physiologic stress, our focus here is on the latter. Our emphasis is on maintaining fuel supply to the brain during the two critical periods in the 24-hour cycle when metabolic stress may be acute (exercise) and/or chronic (during the night fast). These are the two periods in our metabolic lives when the liver may become depleted if not optimally fueled.

Historical Summary of Liver Glycogen - Energy Status Research

In 1963 M Rusek hypothesized that liver glucoreceptors were involved in regulating appetite and feeding response.[110]

In 1984 RL Hanson and team looked at a compound known as 2,5-Anhydro-D-mannitol (2,5-AM), a fructose analogue that inhibits both glycogenolysis and gluconeogenesis, and therefore lowers the energy status of the liver.[111] When injected into the portal vein of mice and rats 2,5-AM stimulates hyperphagia (raised appetite and excess eating).

In the 1990s, Freedman and associates revisited this important physiology.[112] They confirmed the work on 2,5-AM in a published paper which stated: "These findings raise the possibility that *changes in hepatic energy status play a role in satiation as well as in hunger* (emphasis added)."[113]

In 2005, Friedman, *et al* suggest that "Theoretical changes in hepatic energy status could be transmitted to the brain via a neural or humoral route; at present, however, there is evidence only for a neural connection, specifically via vagal afferent neurons."[114]

This latter statement is a bit strange given that in 2002, Jean-Marc Lavoie and his team at Montreal University published the results of an animal study in which they demonstrated that as liver glycogen depletes during exercise, the liver releases a protein known as IGFBP-1.[115] This release is directly proportional to the rate of liver glycogen depletion. It seems that IGFBP-1 is the critical hormonal signal (overlooked by Friedman) warning the brain that trouble is ahead if action is not taken to replenish liver glycogen and maintain fuel supply to the brain during exercise. [More on this in Chapter 7.]

It is known that IGFBP-1 also rises, not unexpectedly, during the night fast.[116] This provides another illustration of the liver's role in warning the brain with regard to its energy status.

Much earlier (1950), WS Bullough of the University of Sheffield and EA Eisa of the Farouk I University, Alexandria had already made a direct connection between liver energy status and recovery physiology. Their study looked at mitosis (or cell division) in the skin of mice and compared cell glycogen levels with that of liver glycogen, which in effect viewed mitosis as an index of recovery. In their comments, they state "It has now been shown that the skin glycogen concentration varies with that of the liver, and from various data available some understanding of the glycogen rhythm may be obtained . . . *In both normal and abnormal conditions a high concentration of glycogen in the skin coincides with a high rate of epidermal mitotic activity, while a low glycogen concentration coincides with low mitotic activity* (emphasis added).[117]

It may seem surprising that the significance of this historic study was missed for such a lengthy time. The connection between liver glycogen plenitude and recovery physiology, attracts little interest in medical and exercise physiology faculties even today.

Melatonin - the Hormone of the Night

Our discussion of restorative sleep would not be complete without mention of melatonin. Melatonin is a naturally occuring hormone secreted from the pineal gland in the brain. It has sometimes been referred to as the "wellness hormone" due to the wide range of healthful effects it facilitates within the human body.

The pineal gland is a small endocrine gland about the size of a pea located in the center of the brain between the two hemispheres. It is often referred to as the "third eye" as light sensitive cells in the retina signal the SCN which in turns relays these circadian signals by way of other brain nuclei, the spinal cord, and the sympathetic nervous system to the pineal gland. The pineal gland secretes melatonin in response to falling light levels, and melatonin regulates the circadian clock. This aspect of the physiogogy of melatonin has resulted in its popular use by those who travel across multiple time zones and by individuals with sleep disorders. However, these uses express only a small portion of the many roles of this hormone.

It is the blue region of the light spectrum that inhibits melatonin release. In recent years, lighting products have been developed that do not emit light in this range with the goal to improve melatonin production even when the lights are on. Light pollution from within and without the home affects most humans throughout the 24-hour cycle.

Humans are diurnal creatures and will function with metabolic efficiency over the night hours, albeit with a certain toll on health. Previously we have commented on the negative impact of shift work on metabolism from poor qualtiy and shortened sleep. Other research has documented a link between increases in certain forms of cancer with a reduction of melatonin observed in shift workers.[118, 119]

Not only is melatonin known for its anticarcinogenic properties,[120] it also is a potent antioxidant. Melatonin is released during exercise, suggestive of a protective role in brain cells when exposed to increased risk of oxidative damage.[121] This amazing hormone also recycles other antioxidant principles, such as vitamin C, so that they may be used again after oxidation of free radicals (known as redox cycling). Melatonin is increasingly recognised as a potent immune system stimulant.[122] This fact relates directly to the role of sleep as a modulator of immune function.

As we have noted above in the opening pages of this chapter, the liver glycogen store is quite small when compared to the total glycogen stores contained in the muscle cells. (The muscle glycogen store has the capacity to store more than ten times the amount of glycogen than can be stored in the liver.) Even when optimally replenished with its full complement of glycogen before bedtime, the liver store may be at risk due to several of the conditions described above. Inadequate liver glycogen means insufficient fuel for the brain during sleep.

Honey consumed before bedtime will result in the formation and release of melatonin by way of the HYMN Cycle described in more detail in Poster No 14 found in Appendix E. By contributing to the release of melatonin during sleep, honey may be characterized as a facilitator of the many healthful benefits associated with this hormone.

Melatonin, Memory, and Metabolic Stress

Melatonin may play a role in improving memory consolidation during REM (rapid eye movement) sleep. A recent study by G. Baydas and team demonstrated that melatonin exerts a modulatory effect in structural remodelling of synaptic connections during memory learning processes during REM sleep.[123] Neural cell adhesion molecules (NCAMS) are members of the immunoglobulin superfamily and are involved in synaptic rearrangements in the mature brain. They play a central role in memory processing particularly during REM sleep, when short term memories are passed from the hippocampus into long term memory maintained in the cortex.

This research has potent implications for learning both in adults and children. As we move further and further away from our relationship with the natural light/dark cycle because of artificial lighting, the impact on our health becomes more and more profound and negative. In addition, electromagnetic waves suppress melatonin production. Millions of children retire to bed with the television set on or a variety of other wave-emitting electronic devices activated. The result is lowered nocturnal melatonin production.

The long term impact of this on learning and health may be discovered in decades to come. However, if melatonin release is the key causal event in growth hormone release and in the activation of recovery physiology, then it may be that not only are our children not recovering during sleep, they are not learning up to their potential during wakefullness. Sleeping in a metabolic and cellular environment bathed in stress hormones due to diminished melatonin release is bound to have ongoing impact of growth physiology and neural development.

In the 2005 paper "Sleepless in America " by Turek and Bass,[124] the authors point out that children are sleeping up to two hours less than required according to the American National Sleep Foundation. Couple this with the Eve Van Cauter study that demonstrated a marked negative change in the metabolic profile of healthy young men after sleep deprivation of four hours a night for only six nights and we have a window into the modern metabolic syndrome, a window into a Dantian metabolic inferno. What health risks can be forecast for millions of our youth who from an early age enter a state of light-driven, electromagnetic wave-disturbed, shortened sleep, all of which contribute to increased metabolic stress every night of their lives?

Sleep and Offline Processing

An American researcher Jonathan Winson has postulated an interesting link between neural cell processing of information during REM sleep and the unconscious mind. During REM sleep the motor system is inhibited. However, the theta waves generated in the brain during this sleep mimic survival processing without the motor activity that typically accompanies it. Winson's hypothesis is based on the concept that this offline processing mimics survival behavior during episodes of fight/flight survival and thus may represent a kind of training for future such episodes. In other words, the information processing required to improve survival options online during a crisis are being rehearsed during REM sleep. This "training" would involve integrating old with new knowledge. The dream, as it is experienced and described, is simply a window for our conscious mind to tune into the process. Winson's perspective is enhanced by other studies that show that post-training increases the intensity of REM sleep.[125]

Honey and Its Role in Sleep, Dreams and Learning

One of the most interesting and common anecdotal feedback responses received from those who consume a tablespoon or two of honey prior to bedtime in order to restock the liver glycogen store is that of increased dream intensity and recall. It may be argued that this pre-bedtime fueling reduces the occurence of metabolic stess and thus improves the intensity of REM sleep. Direct association between honey eaten before bed and REM sleep will require more investigation. We do know that honey improves memory and reduces anxiety when compared to sucrose in animal studies.[126] Honey also reduces metabolic and oxidative stress, both of which affect sleep state and duration.

Acceptance of the hypothesis that honey eaten before bedtime increases the intensity of REM sleep and therefore of improved memory processing leads to a model for improved learning. The logic would argue that liver replenishment prior to bedtime insures restorative sleep, which in turn facilitates offline processing, memory and learning. More research is needed to confirm this simple hypothesis. In the meantime, there is no risk associated with consuming honey before bedtime. Those who have begun this habit may well be ahead of the game in experiencing improved brain function, including improved memory and learning.

It was in 1920 that a noteworthy dream was recorded by the German physiologist, Otto Loewi. Loewi had a vague idea about information transmission by chemicals as opposed to nerves as early as 1903 but was unable to confirm this. Some 17 years later he recorded his experience:

"The night before Easter Sunday of that year I awoke, turned on the light, and jotted down a few notes on a tiny slip of paper. Then I fell asleep again. It occurred to me at 6 o'clock in the morning that during the night I had written down something most important, but I was unable to decipher the scrawl. The next night, at 3 o'clock, the idea returned. It was the design of an experiment to determine whether or not the hypothesis of chemical transmission that I had uttered 17 years ago was correct. I got up immediately, went to the laboratory, and performed a single experiment on a frog's heart according to the nocturnal design."[127]

In any event this iconic and dream-inspired experiment that he carried out earned him the Nobel Prize for Medicine in 1936. Loewi's work became the basis of our knowledge of hormonal information transmissions within nervous tissue and opened a fertile window into the field of molecular physiology. We will never know the status of Otto Loewi's liver glycogen store on that night in 1920, but we do feel entitled to speculate. Perhaps he had a late meal on the night of the second dream, or perhaps he may have had honey with his supper prior to bed. Certainly his REM sleep was intensified on that night. This anecdote suggests that Otto Loewi's dream recall may be included with those of our many other pre-bedtime honey eaters.

What Is Sleep?

Much about sleep continues to be an enigma. We do know when we are and when we are not sleeping. However in spite of a century of research, we are still at a loss to fully explain exactly what sleep is, and what complex purposes may be fulfilled when sleeping. The debate involves a wide range of the entire academic life science spectrum, including the disciplines of neuroscience, endocrinology, psychoneuroendocrinology, psychology, psychiatry, metabolism, physiology, somnology, immunology, and even philosophy.

We know a great deal about the different sleep stages, the various brain waves exhibited during each, and the metabolic environments we may generate during sleep, both positive and negative. We have learned much about what occurs during REM and non-REM sleep.[128] We know that sleep controls modulation of the immune system. We understand the role of sleep in circadian cycles and thermoregulation. We know about the activation of various brain regions during sleep such as the hypothalamus, the hippocampus, the SCN, and which neural populations are involved. Less is known (though much is written) about dreams, what exactly they are and what may be their purpose.

Restorative Sleep and How to Get It

Little has been published about restrorative sleep and recovery physiology and what one may do to optimise recovery physiology during sleep. The principle of optimising recovery by refueling the liver with honey prior to bedtime was first explained in **The Hibernation Diet**. Honey stabilizes blood sugar levels and prevents metabolic stress from occuring. Honey also prompts a small insulin spike which leads to the release of melatonin. Melatonin is responsible for a literal cascade of recovery mechanisms that occur during sleep [See Poster No 14 - Honey, Sleep and the HYMN Cycle in Appendix E].

For individuals habituated by a culture that eats early in the evening and goes to bed late, a tablespoon or two of pure, unprocessed honey[129] prior to bed activates this recovery sleep cycle and insures proper functioning of restorative physiology. Sleep quality will be improved, recovery (fat burning) physiology will be optimized, and the chronic release of adrenal stress hormones resulting in multiple conditions associated with the metabolic syndrome will be inhibited. Those who follow this simple regimen can have confidence in knowing that they are improving their own health state as well as participating in a revolution. As a generation of individuals join in, we will see reductions in the risks for all the diseases associated with the metabolic syndrome including adult and childhood obestiy, diabetes, cardiovascular disease, osteoporosis, gastric ulcers, depression, memory loss and dementia.

Restorative Sleep and the Immune System

The overwhelming urge to sleep is an intuitive and innate response to bouts of sickness. Sleep and immune response are intimately correlated. Each has potent modulatory effects on the other. Some immune factors are powerful sleep inducers, and sleep in turn modulates the immune system. Interleukins, TNF-alpha and interferon gamma rise during the night hours. In general, most inflammatory immune cells and factors are raised during resting metabolism, and in particular at night. The circadian variation in immune response has been confirmed in diurnal rodents that mimic human circadian immune modulation, as opposed to nocturnal rodents that express a reversed circadian phase.

M.V. Leone and others from her Argentinian team published a review of the interaction between sleep and the immune system in 2007.[130] The authors demonstrate that the circadian variation of immune response was optimal during daylight hours and lower during nocturnal hours, suggesting a recovery phase during resting metabolism. Immune system circadian modulation appears to mimic circadian physiology with activity in the diurnal phase and recovery during the nocturnal phase. The authors refer to increased slow wave sleep (SWS) following infection and that administration of bacterial components invoke somnogenic effects, namely increased SWS duration, and decreased REM (rapid eye movement) sleep. The authors also demonstrate feedback interaction between CLOCK genes and the immune system further confirming the link between the light/dark cycle and immune system competence.

In this chapter we have linked liver glycogen status with recovery physiology optimised by consuming honey prior to sleep, and postulate that this link most specifically includes the immune system. This link is confirmed by noting the effects of chronic metabolic stress on immunity. Poor quality and foreshortened sleep impedes normal recovery physiology and results in compromised immune system functioning over time. This expresses itself within the general population and more potently in the athletic community all too frequently as impaired health and increasingly prevalent disease states.

A Nocturnal Wake-up Call

The relationship between the energy or fuel status of the liver and the quality and duration of restorative sleep is one of the most neglected areas of human physiology. Chronic nocturnal metabolic stress can be easily prevented by simply providing adequate fuel for the liver during the night fast. The modern myth that discourages eating before bedtime contributes to this failure to restock the critical liver storehouse with glycogen. *The ultimate outcome from months and years of neglecting to provide fuel for the liver and hence the brain during sleep contributes to a rising tide of related metabolic disorders associated with poor quality sleep.* These disorders include childhood and adult obesity, Type 2 Diabetes, hypertension and cardiovascular disease, immune system malfunction, gastric ulcers and other gastrointestinal disorders, infertility, depression, memory loss, dementias and Alzheimer's disease.

All of these conditions are directly connected to poor liver glycogen status. As the liver supply of glycogen reaches low levels, the "stress" protein IGFBP-1 is released to warn the brain of low fuel status. Insulin-like growth factor-1 (IGF-1)[131] is inhibited and cellular death, rather than cell restoration and recovery, progresses unabated. The brain releases other stress hormones, cortisol and adrenalin in order to produce glucose from muscle protein and insure adequate brain fuel supply. Cortisol is the key hormone associated with metabolic stress.

Another fascinating recent discovery in this unfolding narrative links IGF-1 to an enzyme known as 11 beta-hydroxysteroid dehydrogenase-1 (11beta-HSD-1). This enzyme is found in the liver, adipose (fat) tissue, brain and muscle, the organs and tissues intimately involved in energy homeostasis. It acts in each of these tissues to activate cortisol from its inactive form cortisone. 11beta-HSD-1 has been found to be active in producing intracellular cortisol in conditions of the metabolic syndrome, even when serum cortisol levels are normal. When IGF-1 is inhibited, 11beta-HSD-1 levels are elevated resulting in activation of cortisol within the cells. This intracellular stress is "hidden" and not apparent from monitoring circulating cortisol levels.

This link completes the model for understanding the relationship between the liver glucose/glycogen store, peripheral glucose metabolism in muscle, and the cascade of conditions known as the metabolic syndrome. When liver glycogen is low, IGF-1 is inhibited, intracellular 11beta-HSD-1 activates cortisol which in turn inhibits glucose metabolism and disposal in the peripheral tissues. As intracellular glucose levels become elevated, fat metabolism and disposal is also inhibited due to the inhibition of the fat transporter, CPT, giving additional explanation for the consequences of the metabolic syndrome. It seems counter-intuitive that low levels of glucose in the liver affect metabolism of fats in muscle and contribute to obesity and diabetes, but the connections are clear.

Sleep is an energy driven physiologic process. Regulation of sleep energy status is controlled by the SCN and the hypocretins produced in response to light/dark cycles. When a low energy status or low energy supply in the liver threatens normal brain functioning, the process does not simply shut down as when an automobile runs out of gas. Rather a whole host of activities is initiated by way of hormonal release and/or intracellular activation of cortisol by 11beta-HSD-1. This cascade of activity impairs quality sleep and results in metabolic stress that over time results in the conditions referred to as the metabolic syndrome.

How to Achieve Restorative Sleep and Optimize Recovery Physiology During Rest

Natural honey when ingested just before bedtime will optimally refuel the liver and promote quality sleep. Recovery physiology during the night fast is insured and promoted. Metabolic stress is prevented. Memory processing during REM sleep occurs naturally and leads to improved learning. Honey is an inexpensive, non-pharmacological, revolutionary solution that optimizes human physiology throughout our normal circadian rhythms.

A tablespoon or two of natural honey ingested at bedtime replenishes liver glycogen and modulates the first cascading pathway illustrated below in favor of recovery, restful, restorative, metabolically beneficial sleep. Without optimum liver glycogen, the second cascade prevails resulting in metabolic stress and its multiple associated conditions.

The Sweet Hungarian Rhapsody - The Dawn Phenomenon

The Hungarian Rhapsody No 2 by Franz Liszt is perhaps one of the world's most famous piano compositions. The No 2 is from a set of 19 works and remains the most popular. However it is another famous early morning Hungarian rhapsody that commands our attention in this discussion on sleep, the night fast, recovery physiology, and metabolic stress. This sweet physiological expression is that of raised blood glucose concentration in the morning known in the medical sciences as the "Dawn Phenomenon."

This medical curiosity was discovered by a Hungarian physician, Dr. Michael Somogyi, who pioneered work on insulin. Diabetics are most at risk from this condition because they may record a falsely elevated blood glucose level on awakening and overshoot their morning insulin dose, thus precipitating a rapid and dangerous fall in blood glucose concentration.

This form of metabolic stress is seriously underestimated. Most individuals will experience the "dawn phenomenon" to some extent. For many, the phenomenon is experienced as "morning sickness." Morning sickness is typically associated with pregnancy during the first trimester when the expectant mother is nauseous and unable to eat breakfast. Both mother and fetus have used up the liver glycogen store during the night fast. Glucagon, which causes nausea, and other stress hormones (cortisol and adrenalin) are released to maintain blood glucose concentrations. The early morning result is predictable. Nausea, shakiness, perhaps headaches and a sense of low level agitation confirm that the mother has experienced metabolic stress overnight. Low or high blood glucose levels may result depending on the efficiency of the hormonal response.

Both "morning sickness" and the "dawn phenomenon" are the result of the production and release of counter-regulatory (stress) hormones overnight in order to produce glucose from muscle protein. This rise in glucose from degraded protein needed to fuel the brain may produce an impression of an energy surge, albeit a false one, resulting from a depleted liver. The key to both physiological manifestations is the liver glycogen status during the hours of the night fast.

Honey is the perfect food for replenishing the liver prior to bed, activating recovery physiology overnight and preventing the physiologic effects of the "dawn phenomenon" and "morning sickness."

Both conditions occur in athletes during times of rigorous training. Both may be modified positively by optimal refueling of the liver glycogen store prior to bed. For athletes, refueling prior to exercise is also essential in order to prevent the negative consequences of liver depletion, subsequent stress hormone release and protein degradation.

A Cascading Model for Restorative Sleep versus a Model for The Metabolic Syndrome

A MODEL FOR RESTORATIVE SLEEP
By which
Normal Liver Glycogen Leads to Restorative Sleep & Recovery

- **NORMAL** or high **LIVER GLYCOGEN** levels **INSURE**
  - High levels of free IGF-1 which cause
    - Levels of the enzyme 11beta-HDS-1 to remain low
      - Thus keeping cortisone inactive which results in
        - Lowered metabolic stress allowing

RESTORATIVE SLEEP & RECOVERY
versus

A MODEL FOR THE METABOLIC SYNDROME
By which
Low Liver Glycogen Leads to the Metabolic Syndrome

- **LOW LIVER GLYCOGEN** levels trigger the release of
  - Elevated levels of IGFBP-1 which are associated with
    - Elevated levels of the 11beta-HSD-1 which
      - Activate intracellular cortisone producing
        - Increased metabolic stress which results in
          - Poor Quality Sleep and

THE METABOLIC SYNDROME
Which includes:
- Insulin resistance, fasting hyperglycemia, Type 2 Diabetes mellitus or impaired fasting glucose, impaired glucose tolerance
- Hypertension or elevated blood pressure
- Central obesity (also known as visceral, male-pattern or apple-shaped adiposity), overweight with fat deposits mainly around the waist
- Decreased HDL cholesterol (a risk for heart disease)
- Elevated triglycerides and
- Other associated diseases

6 What Fuel for Which Type of Exercise

Chapter Summary

The choice of exercise - aerobic or anaerobic - depends on the desired outcome one is expecting from an exercise program. Proper fueling for exercise requires an understanding of the physiology involved with both types.

The primary fuel for exercise in humans is glucose. Aerobic exercise does not burn fat to any significant degree. The greater the intensity of exercise, the smaller percentage of fat is burned relative to glucose. Anaerobic exercise is a much more efficient form of exercise when weight loss is the desired outcome.

There are two primary systems for storing glycogen - the liver and the muscle cells. The most significant energy storehouse for exercise and recovery is the liver glycogen store. Fueling both the liver and skeletal muscles should be undertaken before, during, and after exercise, and prior to recovery sleep. The focus should be on fuels not calories.

Optimal fueling is as important during training, as it is for competition. Optimal fueling of both muscles and liver will protect muscle proteins from degradation, and reduce production of adrenal stress hormones. Fructose is critical for selective uptake of glucose by the liver; fructose regulates glucose uptake into the liver. A fructose-based fuel during exercise will increase oxidation and therefore power output during exercise.

Fats are never a limiting factor during exercise, and any attempt to release extra fats during exercise will be counter-productive and promote longer-term negative health consequences. Proteins may be a significant fuel used during exercise, however good fueling protocols must be followed that respect the glycogen supply in the liver.

Both exercise and starvation produce similar physiologic responses in the body in which body fuel stores are quickly exhausted.

Without proper fueling, exercising humans will always activate release of stress hormones. Fueling protocols for exercise must take into account optimum fueling for the liver along with muscles.

Aerobic versus Anaerobic Exercise – Which Is Best

Initiating an exercise program frequently begins with a question. What type of exercise is best? Or rather, what type of exercise is best for me? Though the question is sincere, it is a bit naïve. The question as posed is similar to asking "What kind of vehicle shall I buy?" The answer depends entirely on just where you want to go, how comfortable you want to be in route, and how long you want to take to get there.

Physical exercise comes in many forms. Each form has ardent advocates who will steadfastly argue the benefits of one over the other. Tune into cable TV late at night or on a lazy Saturday morning and you can pick from any number of exercise programs promising immediate rock hard abs, a toned derrière, improved overall fitness, or miraculous weight loss.

Simply put, there really are only two types of exercise from a physiologic standpoint. These are aerobic or anaerobic exercise. Which type of physical exercise is best depends on what you are trying to accomplish by your exercise training.

Aerobic exercise, a term developed by Kenneth Cooper, MD,[132] an exercise physiologist and Colonel Pauline Potts, a physical therapist, means simply exercise requiring oxygen in the body's energy-generating process. Aerobic exercise is performed at various levels of intensity over extended periods of time and includes such activities as walking, running, swimming and cycling.

Initially during aerobic exercise, glycogen from the muscle cells or the liver is broken down to provide glucose for fuel. As glycogen stores are depleted, fat metabolism is initiated to provide energy. However the switch to fat as fuel is a slow process and is accompanied by a decline in performance level. The depletion of glycogen stores and the switch to fat as fuel is a major cause of what marathon runners call "hitting the wall."

Aerobic exercise produces both health and performance benefits. Among these are:

- Improved cardiopulmonary capacity and function
- Increased cardiac output and improved pumping efficiency
- Improved muscle toning throughout the body which improves circulation and reduces blood pressure
- Improved oxygen transport via increase in total red blood cells and hemoglobin levels
- Reductions in the risk of osteoporosis
- Increased storage and utilization of both glycogen and fats in muscles which allows increased endurance
- Improved circulation through muscles from new blood vessel formation

- Earlier activation of aerobic metabolism in muscles and improved ability to burn fats
- Enhanced speed of recovery from intense exercise

Anaerobic exercise, sometimes referred to as *resistance exercise*, does not require oxygen to generate energy for the body's muscles. There are two types of energy sources used in anaerobic exercise depending on the duration of the activity. For bursts of activity lasting up to thirty seconds, the body relies on creatine phosphate, a fuel source synthesized in the liver and carried to the muscle cells where it is stored. After thirty seconds, muscle cells must depend on lactic acid for energy. The metabolic cycle of lactic acid, also known as anaerobic glycolysis, uses glucose or glycogen in the absence of oxygen. This system can function for up to two minutes in trained muscles. However, it is an inefficient use of glucose and produces by-products that are detrimental to muscle function. For exercise lasting more than two minutes, the body must revert to aerobic energy for its fuel needs.

If you are trying to increase your body's fat burning potential, then resistance exercise is best. If you are trying to increase your muscle mass and tone, as in strength and weight training, then resistance exercise is again the only choice. Resistance exercise is used by athletes in non-endurance sports to build powerful muscles. Body builders use this form of exercise to build muscle mass. Muscles trained under anaerobic conditions develop quite differently. The result leads to greater performance in short episodes of high intensity activities.

Contrary to conventional wisdom especially among recreational and professional athletes, trainers and most health professionals, *the one thing that aerobic exercise does not do is burn fat to any large percentage*. In fact the more intense the aerobic exercise, the smaller the percentage of fat one burns as fuel. Aerobic exercise burns primarily glucose. The more intense the aerobic exercise, the greater the demand for glucose for energy.

Table 1. Results of Aerobic versus Anaerobic Exercise which follows summarizes the best type of exercise for the desired outcome. Of course there are overlapping benefits between both types of exercise, but generally the result or outcome of any exercise program can be predetermined by one's choice of aerobic or anaerobic exercise.

Table 2. Percentages of Glucose / Fat Burned versus Level of Exercise compares the amount of glucose and fat burned during various levels of exercise. During awake but sedentary non-exercising times of the day, our body's metabolic systems are tuned to burn about 50% fat and 50% glucose. During mild aerobic exercise like walking or slow bicycle riding, the percentage of glucose burned increases to between 60% and 70%. The percentage of glucose burned increases to around 80% during moderate exercise. During intense aerobic exercise, our bodies burn up to 90% glucose for as long as the glycogen stores in our muscles hold out. In other words, the more intense the aerobic exercise, the less fat we burn during the time that we are exercising.

It is during rest or recovery periods that we burn more fat, especially when our muscles are toned and fit with moderate frequent resistance exercise. It must be noted that of the total fat burned during exercise, only half of it comes from adipose or fat stores. The other half is from fat stored as triglycerides in muscle cells.

Table 1. Results of Aerobic versus Anaerobic Exercise

Desired Outcome or Result	Type of Exercise
Cardiovascular fitness	Aerobic
Improved cardiopulmonary function	Aerobic
Endurance training	Aerobic
Increased cardiac output	Aerobic
Improved circulation	Aerobic
Fat burning during recovery or rest	Anaerobic or Resistance
Increased muscle tone	Anaerobic or Resistance
Increased power or strength	Anaerobic or Resistance
Increased muscle mass	Anaerobic or Resistance

Table 2. Percentages of Glucose / Fat Burned versus Level of Exercise

Level of Exercise	Percentage of Glucose or Glycogen Burned	Percentage of Fat Burned
Sedentary or at Rest	40 to 50%	50 to 60%
Mild Aerobic (Walking, slow bike riding)	60 to 70%	30 to 40%
Moderate Aerobic (elliptical trainer, jogging, swimming)	~ 80%	~20%
Intense Aerobic (Running, rowing)	90%	~10%

Oxygen - The Currency for Life

If glucose or glycogen is the primary fuel for the body, then oxygen can be likened to the currency with which it trades. Oxygen is the primary currency that powers the body's energy transactions. Oxidation is the reaction fueling aerobic metabolism. Most of our waking hours are spent in the portion of our energy cycle that depends on oxygen.

When you overspend your bank account, the bank says you are overdrawn. You are in a deficit situation financially. In a similar way, during intense exercise, it is possible to exceed your body's oxygen carrying capacity. At that point, you begin to accumulate "oxygen debt." That term was used for decades and aptly described what was occurring in our systems. Now we refer to this as excess post-exercise oxygen consumption or EPOC. (Oxygen debt was easier . . .)

Just as your bank may impose an overdraft limit on your deficit spending, your body has a limit on the oxygen debt that can be accumulated. With training, you can increase the amount of oxygen debt that you can accumulate before you collapse. Trained athletes increase the oxygen carrying capacity of the blood by increasing the efficiency of the heart pump, the cardiopulmonary circulation and by increasing the amount of hemoglobin that is contained in their red blood cells. Sometimes they do this by training at high altitudes where lower oxygen levels in the atmosphere stimulate more hemoglobin production. More hemoglobin means more ability to carry oxygen to the muscles, heart, kidneys and other tissues.

Anaerobic Metabolism and EPOC

Anaerobic training increases the number of mitochondria within each muscle cell. A multiplied number of miniature fuel cells within each muscle cell allows the process of anaerobic metabolism to create high level power output over short periods of time, at levels aerobic metabolism cannot reach. The cost of this type of output is so great that it may be maintained only over very short periods of time, up to a maximum of around two minutes as stated above. Anaerobic exercise uses only glucose and little or no fat. The fats that are used during such exercise are utilized for basic metabolic functions, not for contracting muscles.

During the anaerobic breakdown of glucose (through pyruvate) only two units of adenosine-5'-triphosphate (ATP)[133] are created for energy use and for this reason, anaerobic metabolism of glucose is highly inefficient. When glucose is metabolized aerobically (with oxygen), the output is around 38 units of ATP.

Fats cannot be metabolized anaerobically. They require oxygen in order to be converted to energy. Glucose alone is used to power anaerobic exercise.

Only glucose provides the necessary level of energy output to drive anaerobic exercise forward.

During periods of EPOC, increased amounts of oxygen are being used. Fuels are also being metabolized above the normal basic metabolic rate. The primary fuel burned during this recovery period is fat. Sustained aerobic exercise also contributes to some oxygen debt or EPOC, but not to the degree that results from anaerobic exercise. For this reason, exercisers desirous of achieving weight (fat) loss should include anaerobic exercise as part of their exercise regime.

Energy Output of Aerobic versus Anaerobic Metabolism Compared

Aerobic Metabolism & Glycolysis

1. Glucose enters the muscle cell by way of a protein transport system known as glut-2
2. Glucose is phosphorylated (a phosphate ion is attached) and becomes glucose-6-phosphate
3. Oxidative phosphorylation produces pyruvate yielding a net of two ATP molecules
4. Oxidative decarboxylation of pyruvate yields another six ATP molecules
5. When oxygen is present, pyruvate produces acetyl-CoA
6. Acetyl-CoA molecules are metabolized within the mitochondria via the Krebs cycle to produce water and CO_2

The complete cycle produces a total theoretical yield of 36-38 ATP molecules with an actual net yield closer to 30 ATP molecules.

Compared to Anaerobic Metabolism

Without oxygen, pyruvate is not transported into the mitochondria but stays in the cytoplasm where it is converted to lactic acid. Lactic acid is used for brief high-energy outputs such as required in sprinting or weight lifting. The energy yield from one glucose molecule is only 2 ATP molecules compared to the 30 to 38 ATP molecules.

Thus, the amount of energy released as ATP during aerobic respiration is 15 to 19 times greater than in anaerobic respiration.

From this point of view aerobic respiration is more efficient than anaerobic respiration.

Anaerobic Exercise and Weight Loss

Because anaerobic metabolism does not use fats for fuel during the anaerobic exercise period, those whose primary goal is to lose weight do not typically think to include this type of exercise in their regimen. But in fact, *anaerobic or resistance exercise is actually a much more efficient form of exercise for weight loss than is aerobic exercise.* This may seem counter-intuitive to many who spend hours on the treadmill in hopes of dropping a few pounds.

As indicated above, aerobic exercise does not primarily burn fat. The more intense the aerobic effort, the less percentage of fat burned for energy. Even though anaerobic or resistance exercise burns only glucose (and *no* fat), the real payoff occurs during the post-exercise rest period and during recovery sleep. Anaerobic exercise causes muscle trauma and damage by free radical buildup within the muscle cells, therefore requiring increased fuel resources to drive recovery physiology. *The energy used to fuel recovery physiology is exclusively fat burning physiology.* In as little as 15 minutes of anaerobic effort, muscle failure will occur. However, this muscle cell fatigue is sufficient to stimulate repair during periods of restorative sleep and recovery physiology, given of course, that the liver is fueled prior to rest or bedtime.

As stated throughout this book, honey is the best food to selectively restock the liver glycogen energy store before rest. Honey provides the correct balance of glucose and fructose to the liver allowing for optimum glycogen formation without added digestive burden late in the evening.

The Partition and Selection of Fuels Used During Exercise

Many health professionals, trainers as well as most professional and recreational athletes, are not aware of the partition and selection of fuels utilized by the body during exercise. As shown above in **Table 2. Percentages of Glucose and Fat Burned according to Level of Exercise**, the amount of fat burned is inversely proportionate to the intensity level of exercise. In other words, as exercise intensity increases, the percentage of fat burned for fuel decreases.

When fuel stores, particularly the liver glycogen store, are not maintained optimally, proteins are degraded and transported to the liver where they are converted to glucose in a process known as gluconeogenesis. During prolonged exercise during which muscle glycogen is depleted, muscle proteins become the primary source for this glucose. The same rule of physiology applies in both cases. Further, the more intense the level of exercise, the greater the percentage of glucose versus fatty acids is consumed or burned as fuel.

We may refer to this relationship as the **Law of Exercise Intensity**. This law states the governing principle controlling the relative proportions of glucose and fats used for fuel during any exercise protocol, regardless of the source of glucose. This **Law of Exercise Intensity** may be formally stated thus:

> *The absolute work rate during exercise determines the total quantity of fuel used, while relative exercise intensity determines the proportions of glucose and fats oxidized in contracting muscles.*

The law may be posed in another way. During exercise, the total work output will determine the total quantity of calories burned. However, the exercise intensity determines or defines the source of the fuel used for this work, whether glucose or fats. The total work output will never determine the kind of fuel burned or its source. This critical measure or ratio is *always* determined by the intensity of exercise, relative to maximum intensity, as laid out in Table 2 above.

This distinction is important because training manuals and diet and exercise literature tend to refer to the amount of calories consumed in various exercise protocols, but fail to focus on the source for these calories. Consider the following from the book "No Carbs After 5pm Diet" by Joanna Hall, one of the leading United Kingdom fitness, diet and lifestyle experts, and a graduate in sports science:

> "Also known as the carb curfew diet, this plan maintains that cutting carbs after 5pm helps cut calories without you having to try too hard. Ultimately, this lowers your overall calorie intake for the day so you lose weight. In addition, eating slightly more protein will help you to stay fuller for longer and cutting carbs can help you feel less bloated."[134]

This focus on calories, without any discussion of what these carbs are or from where they are sourced, is an excellent illustration of the blindness of many exercise physiologists to the importance of the liver glycogen stores before and during exercise. In the above book title's example, no carbs will be consumed after 5:00 PM. Even if one can assume, in this case, that the unfortunate dieter did manage to have a glycogen stocked liver after an early evening meal (such is unlikely given such a restricted diet), he will most certainly enter a period of metabolic stress prior to or early on during the eight hours of the night fast and remain in this state of stressed physiology for the duration of sleep.

A significant portion of the carbohydrates burned by this poor misinformed fellow during his repeated periods of metabolic stress will probably be from muscle proteins, degraded to make glucose to maintain fuel supply for the brain. The result of this chronic overproduction of adrenal stress hormones results in increased risk of all the adrenal driven diseases, including heart disease and diabetes. Any benefits accruing from any exercise protocol undertaken by this individual intended to result in weight loss will simply be cancelled out by the metabolic stress induced by stress physiology during the night. Initial weight loss will consist mainly of loss of muscle protein and water. It is unlikely that this weight loss will be maintained, primarily because as the adrenal hormones increase metabolic stress, orexigenic (appetite increasing) hormones are released. Furthermore, although some of the protein consumed before 5 PM may be used to replenish the liver, this is not an optimal outcome and will result in an increase in the release of glucagon, a hormone associated with low liver glycogen status.

Calorie Fetishism

This type of loose calorie thinking is endemic in the dietary world, and usually results in loss of lean muscle tissue, increased appetite and ultimately a failure to maintain the diet regime, not to mention the ill health that it may bring in its wake. It would not be unreasonable to describe this type of thinking as a form of "**calorie fetishism**."

Focus on Fuels, Not Calories

It is vitally important in all exercise (and diet protocols) to be aware of exactly what fuels are used, when they are used, and from where they are sourced. Simply "counting calories" or "counting carbs" as many nutritionists and dietary counselors advise is not enough. In other words one must focus on the *partition and selection* of fuels, both at rest and during exercise.

Though much has been included about honey in Chapters 1 through 3, we underscore again the role of honey in optimizing recovery within the context of these important metabolic concepts. Honey is both an excellent energy fuel for exercise and a food that may be used to optimize recovery physiology by optimally fueling liver glycogen, the key glycogen store for both exercise and recovery.

The Liver Glycogen Store

Herein we place great emphasis on the liver glycogen store as opposed to muscle glycogen, and on the two fat stores, muscle fat and adipose fat. There are good reasons for this emphasis on liver glycogen. First of all, muscle glycogen has been very well researched and discussed in great detail in sports and exercise fueling literature since the 1960's. Every serious athlete is aware of how and when to fuel muscles before, during and after exercise. This is certainly not the case with the liver glycogen store. Secondly, fats are rarely, if ever, a limiting factor during exercise except in very extreme situations. Fats are available for energy in most every active situation. Usually, there is much more fat available than can or will be utilized. Excess and unused fat in the circulation is simply returned to the fat stores in muscle and adipose tissue. During resting meatbolism some 70% of circulating fatty acids are returned to storage.[135] During moderate exercise some 25% of circulating fatty acids are returned to storage and in the post exercise period, up to 90% of circulating fatty acids are returned to storage.[136]

Athletes and coaches are almost universally "liver blind." Therefore we will focus on this energy storehouse at the expense of the others. We will describe the role of fructose from honey in regulating this store, and finally how **honey** may be used to optimize this store during exercise and recovery.

Two Fuel Storage Systems

In Chapter 2, we discussed the three primary fuels used in human physiology - carbohydrates (glucose or glycogen), fats (fatty acids) and proteins (amino acids, used largely as reserve fuel). We also introduced the two fuel storage systems for glucose, the primary fuel used during exercise. These storage systems are the ***dual glucose storehouses*** found in ***muscle tissue*** and the ***liver***. Glucose is stored in the muscles and the liver as glycogen, a polysaccharide consisting of long chains of attached glucose molecules.

Muscle glycogen is exclusively reserved for use by contracting muscles during locomotion or exercise and is not available for use by other organs or tissues. This is a very important aspect of muscle glycogen metabolism. When glucose is in short supply, as during prolonged exercise or during a period of fasting, other tissues may not access muscle glycogen. It is reserved only for the use of the muscle cells.

Liver glycogen, on the other hand is available as fuel for many organs/ tissues in the body providing glucose for the heart, kidneys, red blood cells and of course, most importantly, the brain. It also performs a number of important physiologic functions as well, such as acting as an appetite and weight control regulator. In contrast, muscle glycogen performs only one essential function, that of providing glucose to create ATP, the energy force used by contracting muscles during any type of physical exercise. Liver glycogen, by contrast, is a shared fuel resource.

This distinction between muscle and liver glycogen stores is of vital importance as the glycogen from these two sources performs very different physiological roles. In the late 19th century and during the first half of the 20th century there was widespread debate and discussion as to what exactly were the important fuels used during exercise. Most of the scientific debate during that time focused on the role of proteins. That focus continued until later in the 20th century. During the late 1960's, Hultman and his associates described the role of ***muscle glycogen*** during endurance exercise.[137] From that time until now, sports literature has focused on fueling this glycogen store, before, during and after exercise. At the same time, there has been an almost complete lack of interest in the critical role of liver glycogen. Liver glycogen is rarely referred to in exercise physiology and sporting literature, and if it is, the references are slight and in passing, with the emphasis being placed on its role in fueling muscles.

Liver Blindness Can Lead to Metabolic Crisis

When one considers that liver glycogen is the most critical fuel store in human physiology by virtue of the fact that it is the *only* fuel store for the brain, it is curious how this has been ignored. In a recent edition of a booklet "Body Fuel: Food for Sport," by the organization Peak Performance, liver glycogen is referred to *exactly once*.[138] Neither is there any explanation of liver glycogen capacity, nor of the role of liver glycogen at rest, during exercise, during the night fast, or of its vital role during recovery physiology. In other words, this otherwise excellent and informative publication fails to take into account the fuel demand of the brain, the fuel capacity of the liver, the rate of liver depletion during resting metabolism, the rate of glycogen depletion during exercise or of the role of liver glycogen during recovery. These are critical and not insignificant oversights.

This single though not isolated illustration serves to underscore a major conundrum that exists in exercise physiology literature. How is it that the most critical situation in human metabolism - that of maintaining fuel supply to the brain during exercise - is ignored? Contracting muscles are competing at an accelerated rate for the same supply of glucose from the circulation as the brain. This focus would seem to take precedence over all other factors discussed within the context of exercise physiology and metabolism.

This situation is analogous to a race car engineer providing for the fuel requirements of a high performance racing automobile by way of a dual system in which the primary propulsion system (the drive train) competes for or "steals" from the fuel supply required to operate the control, command and governing systems, such that they are prevented from functioning. Any designer of such a model would have a very short career.

When talking with young undergraduates and graduates from sports' science faculties, it very quickly becomes clear that they have little or no concept of the role of liver glycogen. Nor do most exercise physiologists know how the liver may be optimally fueled for exercise and for recovery, never mind the essential role of fructose in all of this. Our repeated experience over several years confirms that this is the case, giving understanding to just why athletes and their coaches are equally "liver blind." It is this blindness that explains why athletes suffer, in many cases, from poor exercise training, poor performance, poor recovery and in the longer term, compromised health, as a result of chronic overproduction of adrenal hormones directly resulting from poor liver fueling. "Liver blindness" is not a disease as such, but it may be termed *a social or cultural disorder*, which begins in the medical faculties of our universities, infects other health, nutrition and dietetics institutions, and impacts the sport science faculties with significant negative consequences.

It is important to note again the emphasis on two separate and distinct fuel storage systems, the liver/brain fuel system and the muscle fuel system. Resting metabolism during the postprandial period (the period of up to two hours after a meal) depends primarily on glucose and fatty acids present in the circulation for fuel. During this period, the liver may also release some 10 grams of glucose per hour into the general circulation, 6.5 grams going to the brain and the remaining 3.5 grams to the heart, kidneys, red blood cells and other tissues. The total amount of glucose (glycogen) utilized as fuel during rest is small compared to the amount of fats burned. The great majority of energy used at rest is provided by fatty acids delivered to tissues by the circulating blood with most of this fuel being consumed by the muscles undergoing repair and recovery.

In contrast, during exercise, contracting muscles utilize the two onsite intracellular stores, muscle fats (triglycerides) and muscle glycogen. However, they also utilize circulating glucose sourced from liver glycogen and fatty acids sourced from body (adipose) fat stores. During exercise therefore, both the liver/brain system and the muscle system depend on glucose from circulating blood. In this sense, both muscles and the brain are competing for the same fuel – glucose sourced from liver glycogen.

It is necessary at this critical juncture to point out that in human physiology, the two systems seem to exist in a state of competitive conflict. If liver glycogen runs dangerously low, the brain requirement overrides that of muscle (and indeed all other tissues) activating the release of metabolic stress hormones as a way of prompting the synthesis of glucose from muscle protein. Athletes experience this situation when blood glucose falls dangerously low (hypoglycemia). As a last resort, the brain will activate a neuro-muscular collapse to forestall the onset of a coma. If the situation is not rapidly resolved, a coma will result.

Many readers will remember how Paula Radcliffe, the world's leading marathon athlete, collapsed during the Athens Olympic Marathon. The condition was blamed on heat exhaustion. This is unlikely in such a trained athlete used to such conditions. It seems much more likely that her liver glycogen rate of depletion was raised beyond her normal rate due to the heat and hilly terrain. She was not degrading muscle protein sufficiently fast enough to create new glucose, maintain blood glucose stability and provide adequate fuel supply to the brain.

Liver Blindness in Sports

"Liver blindness" is universal in modern sports. Tragically, athletes pay a heavy price in long term health consequences for failing to consider the liver during training, performance, and recovery. The liver is the key organ in metabolism during exercise and recovery, although one would find it hard to appreciate this critical fact from reading any book on nutrition and fueling for exercise.

Once exercise is initiated, the liver begins to deplete its glycogen stores. As depletion continues, a stress protein, IGFBP-1 is released from the liver to warn the brain of diminishing liver glycogen levels. This protein inhibits IGF-,1 the key insulinic factor driving glucose into muscle. Fueling the liver and maintaining an adequate liver glycogen store allows for free IGF-1, which in turn allows for increased glucose delivery into muscle, increased glucose oxidation, and therefore increased power output.

Release of IGFBP-1 as the liver is being depleted of glycogen is the signal for increased release of stress hormones causing degradation of muscle protein necessary to produce glucose required to refuel the liver. Liver glycogen is required to maintain fuel supply to the brain which is always at risk during exercise. Chronic release of stress hormones during exercise and during overnight recovery results in long term increased health risks for many conditions in athletes such as motor neurone disease, diabetes, and cardiovascular disease.

The ingestion of fructose in the correct ratio with glucose is the key to proper liver fueling for exercise and for optimum recovery during rest. Two ounces of natural honey, for example, or a commercial product such as *IsoTorque+* provide this proper ratio. The benefits of fructose-based fuels during exercise and performance include:

- Improved training gains
- Improved power output
- Improved mental state
- Improved performance
- Improved recovery
- Improved long term health, and
- Reduced risk for chronic metabolic disease

In situations like this, the brain simply activates a deep and protective fatigue state, regardless of muscle glycogen level. Running low on liver glycogen is a life (brain) threatening condition, and since the brain requirement for glucose always overrides all other requirements, the brain will act long before this potential catastrophe occurs, and arrange for fuel backup from degraded muscle proteins.

There is a powerful lesson in this for all endurance athletes. Running low on muscle glycogen is not a life threatening condition. Contracting muscles may also use fats and still function. However, output will drop to around 50% of potential of capacity. *Running low in liver glycogen is potentially life threatening as it directly impacts brain function.*

Liver Glycogen and How It Signals the Brain

Most of the early scientific work on liver glycogen was carried out in the 1930's and 1940's. Subsequently, serious scientific interest in this organ's fuel store became quite unfashionable. Textbooks on physiology and biochemistry provided detailed descriptions of the pathway known as gluconeogenesis, the creation of glucose from non-carbohydrate sources, a process that occurs mainly in the liver. Beyond that, the dynamic supply of energy from the liver to muscle and especially the brain whose glucose demand is at a premium aroused little interest.

During our research on liver glycogen and its role in exercise and recovery, we surmised that when liver glycogen was low, a situation placing the brain in acute metabolic danger if no backup fuel was available, the liver may release some signal to warn the brain that liver glycogen is low and that action is required urgently to create new glucose to replenish liver glycogen. Such an early warning signal is indeed available.

Insulin-like Growth Factor Binding Protein-1 (IGFBP-1) - Its Role during Exercise

Some have believed that the brain monitored the levels of circulating blood glucose as a way of indicating fuel status, perhaps using the enzyme glucokinase found in the hypothalamus of the brain. We do know that glucokinase in the hypothalamus works in a regulatory manner in response to rising or falling levels of blood glucose. However, this measure is a poor indicator of the actual fuel status of the liver glycogen store. In this sense, blood glucose is a poor indicator of the available fuel for the critical liver/ brain-fueling axis.

Think of it this way. When you turn on the water tap in the morning and the pressure is good, what indication do you have of the amount of water remaining in the water tower or reservoir? Can you tell if the reservoir is nine-tenths full or nearly empty? No, this information requires the action of someone from the water department to give adequate forewarning of water shortages.

This analogy is descriptive of the situation occurring in the brain with regard to liver glycogen stores. Circulating blood glucose levels cannot inform the brain as to an impending fuel shortage due to low liver glycogen levels. The adrenal hormones released during exercise act as **a metabolic response** to low liver glycogen, but they do not act as a **signal** warning the brain of trouble ahead.

An initial search of the literature for such a signal provided no answer. However, recent work by Jean-Marc Lavoie and his team in Montreal University has focused on a protein known as Insulin-like Growth Factor Binding Protein-1 (IGFBP-1). They found that during exercise IGFBP-1 is released from the liver. This release is inversely proportional to liver glycogen plenitude and is **independent** of blood glucose and insulin levels.[139] [See the text box that follows on page 88 entitled **Insulin-like Growth Factor Binding Proteins and the IGF Axis** for a more detailed description of the role of IGFBP-1.]

It is important to note again that the release of IGFBP-1 is independent of blood glucose concentrations. Liver depletion may be occurring even when blood glucose is apparently stable. If IGFBP-1 levels were linked only to blood glucose levels, liver depletion would not initiate a warning signal to the brain indicating an impending fuel shortage. Following the water analogy, water is flowing from the tap, yet the reservoir is nearly dry.

Insulin-like Growth Factor Binding Proteins (IGFBPs) and the IGF Axis

There are actually several insulin-like growth factors (IGFs), ten of them to be exact, two cell-surface receptors, two bonding molecules and a family of six IGF binding proteins along with their associated IGFBP degrading enzymes.[140] The IGF binding proteins are known as IGFBP 1-6. The IGFs are a series of growth and recovery factors with powerful pro-insulin activity. Their role is to rapidly drive glucose into muscle tissue.[141] This response is emerging as a critical alarm signal warning the brain of an impending metabolic catastrophe.

The key factor during exercise is IGF-1. When and if liver glycogen is low, IGF-1 will be inhibited by IGFBP-1 resulting in less glucose entering muscles. IGFBP-1 will bind IGF-1, thus inhibiting its action, reducing glucose uptake by contracting muscles. Glucose is kept in the circulation thereby maintaining blood glucose concentration and protecting liver glycogen levels.

In a sense, IGFBP-1 is a classic stress factor released during periods when glucose supply is at a premium. In addition to this, IGFBP-1 functions as a clever protein providing a metabolic signal to warn the brain of impending fuel shortage. Its release is associated with release of other stress hormones, glucagon, adrenaline and cortisol. Chronic release of IGFBP-1 is now emerging as a marker for Type 2 Diabetes, which is not surprising insofar as cortisol is the other hormone most often associated with insulin resistance. IGFBP-1 levels also rise during the night fast.[142, 143] IGFBP-1 has also has been shown to be elevated during space flight, a form of physiologic stress associated with chronic increased metabolic stress.[144]

IGFBP-1, Liver Glycogen, Glucokinase and Glucose-Based Sports Drinks

In Chapter 2, we described how fructose from honey liberates the glucose enzyme, glucokinase, from the liver cell nucleus, facilitating glucose uptake into the liver and formation of liver glycogen. [See the Fructose Paradox on page 15.]

A significant corollary to that principle is that during exercise, glucokinase, the glucose enzyme, under the influence of adrenalin, will remain locked in the liver cell nucleus. It will not be available to facilitate glucose uptake. This is one of the key principles elaborated in **The Hibernation Diet.**[145]

When glucokinase is not available to facilitate glucose uptake, the formation of liver glycogen during exercise is difficult, if not impossible. As most sport energy drinks are based on glucose or glucose polymers, little or none of this fuel is available for the liver - glucose simply passes through the portal circulation of the liver, entering the general circulation.

However, as sustained exercise further depletes liver glycogen stores, IGFBP-1 is released. IGFBP-1 binds with IGF-1 blocking its action and inhibiting glucose uptake by contracting muscles in an attempt to maintain blood glucose concentration and protect liver glycogen. IGFBP-1 also signals the brain that its fuel supply is getting low. The brain acts by releasing metabolic stress hormones, cortisol and adrenaline, resulting in increased metabolic stress and degradation of muscle proteins to form glucose.

Jean-Marc Lavoie has beautifully confirmed this in his work.[146] He exercised fed rats until they exhibited significant loss of liver glycogen. He then exercised half-fed rats and these rats also exhibited dangerously low levels of liver glycogen. He then exercised the half-fed rats, but infused them with glucose throughout the exercise protocol. These glucose-infused rats also exhibited the same loss of liver glycogen and dangerously low levels of liver glycogen as the non-infused rats.

The Need for Fructose

The clear explanation for this observation by Lavoie is that glucokinase was not available to facilitate glucose uptake into the liver. In spite of increased circulating glucose in the infused group of exercising animals, **no increase in liver glycogen** was recorded. This is a quite stunning confirmation of the necessity of providing a **fructose**-based fuel during all exercise protocols as a means of protecting the fuel supply to the brain and reducing metabolic stress.

Blood Sugar and Homeostasis

Living tissue consists of millions of structural and active principles that must be maintained in a controlled and stable (mostly intracellular) environment, so that these highly reactive and labile principles are not damaged by rapid internal or environmental changes such as temperature, hydration, salinity, acidity, toxicity, and so on. Slight alterations in these parameters may have dramatic and damaging effects on physiology, and therefore the human body utilizes a large number of finely tuned metabolic mechanisms to maintain stability, as and when, this may be disrupted. This stability is known as homeostasis, or balance, and was discovered by Claude Barnard. (Barnard, it happens, was also the discoverer of liver glycogen, the most important fuel store for maintaining just that balance in human physiology.)[147, 148]

The gold standard marker for homeostasis in the human system is the measurement of the blood glucose concentration. Blood glucose is maintained within a very strict and narrow range. This normal range is between 70 and 110 mg/dl (milligrams per deciliter), sometimes referred to as 70 to 110 mg%. If blood glucose concentration rises above 110 mg%, the condition is known as hyperglycemia. If it drops below 70%, it is known as hypoglycemia. Both conditions are potentially dangerous if not tightly monitored and corrected. This monitoring and correction involves a wide range of physiological mechanisms active in the liver, pancreas, gut, and hypothalamus which feed back signals to the brain and release of hormone cascades that respond rapidly to changes in blood glucose homeostasis.

Whenever the human body is faced with an acute metabolic challenge, such as the variations in blood glucose referred to above, the overriding physiological requirement is to maintain adequate and stable glucose supply to the brain by preventing a rapid fall in blood glucose. Resources are mobilized at the expense of all other metabolic requirements to ensure this takes place.

Diabetes Mellitus and Hypoglycemia

Diabetes mellitus is the condition associated with a high level of blood glucose concentration (high blood sugar). Type 1 diabetes is characterized by loss of the insulin-producing beta cells of the islets of Langerhans in the pancreas resulting in a deficiency of insulin. Type 2 Diabetes (sometimes called adult onset diabetes) is due to insulin resistance or reduced insulin sensitivity, combined with reduced insulin secretion. Insulin is the hormone responsible for driving circulating blood glucose into the cells where it can be used as fuel or stored as fat for later use. When insulin is either deficient or ineffective, blood glucose levels rise and may remain elevated.

Hypoglycemia or low blood sugar is less well known but many people do suffer from this condition on a regular basis. The clinical diagnosis in symptomatic individuals is called "functional hypoglycemia." The condition is transient, lasting only a few minutes as the body is quick to respond to low or falling blood sugar levels with the production of adrenal hormones which mobilize protein (mostly from the muscles) for conversion to glucose.

Exercise and Starvation - Similar Challenges for the Body

Two particular conditions that present the body with a significant metabolic challenge are exercise and starvation. Both produce similar physiologic responses, such that we may learn from comparing and contrasting the two. During starvation, body fuel stores are quickly exhausted. Then body tissues are raided to create fuel for the maintenance of life. Exercise is in many ways (although not all) similar to starvation. Fuels are being rapidly used up, and if not replenished, body tissues are degraded to provide backup fuel.

Exercise as a Form of First Stage Starvation

Exercise presents the human body with a series of metabolic challenges that, it seems fair to state, may be life threatening. Most fit young athletes, who train on a daily basis, may view a statement such as this with skepticism, but a little reflection on the dynamics of exercise and the fuels used may place this in its correct metabolic context.

Starvation on the other hand may be described in three distinct stages. **Stage 1** involves resources being mobilized to maintain blood glucose concentration and fuel supply to the brain. This occurs only after some hours without food. This stage is dominated by stress physiology in which non-essential proteins are degraded (mainly from muscle and from the gut), taken to the liver in the form of amino acids, and converted to glucose (the process of gluconeogenesis).

This stage highlights one of the most widely misunderstood aspects of human physiology, that of release of adrenal hormones known throughout the literature of physiology as *"fight or flight"* hormones. Adrenal hormones are indeed released during fight or flight episodes, but they serve to **inhibit muscle uptake of glucose**! It is this critical metabolic function that is often overlooked. Adrenal hormones (primarily cortisol) are released to make glucose available (from muscle protein) to the circulation during periods when contracting muscles are extracting this glucose. It is also during this time that the brain is placed in metabolic danger. The glucose produced from protein via the effects of cortisol also serves to fuel the brain. Therefore it is **incorrect** to describe these hormones as only *fight or flight* hormones. They are in fact **neuro-protective** hormones.

Chronic, repetitive overproduction of these hormones, also known as glucocorticoids (cortisol and adrenalin), leads to insulin resistance by virtue of the fact that these hormones are doing their physiological duty very efficiently – they inhibit the cellular uptake of glucose! After several days, the cannibalizing assault on proteins to make glucose enters a more dangerous phase. More essential proteins, such as cardiac muscle and other enzyme systems may be at risk.

This first stage of starvation, which is dominated by a stressed physiology, is the stage similar to exercise. Exercising humans will always activate release of stress hormones if they are not careful. To minimized this release, it is necessary to fuel the liver, along with muscles.

Stage 2 begins with the onset of ketosis, a process by which fats are taken to the liver and converted into ketones, as described in Chapter 2. This stage is characterized by the lack of requirement for adrenal hormone release and resembles the physiology of hibernation and bird migration, where the brain is fueled by ketones while essential proteins are protected. Exercise in humans **can never directly activate ketosis,** and any ketones produced are not significant in quantity.

Stage 3 starvation is reached when fat stores run low, and the body will return to proteins as a source of fuel. This is the end game, and death is close.

Exercise As an Aggressive Form of Starvation

During starvation most people are in a resting physiological state, a state of lethargy that would not encourage physical activity, and therefore depletion of energy stores will take place more slowly than during exercise. It is instructive therefore, to consider exercise as a specialized form of accelerated starvation, and potentially more toxic in the short term.

During exercise, energy stores are being rapidly depleted as if in a state of aggressive starvation. If those energy stores are not rapidly replenished, the body must mobilize all resources to maintain the level of physical output, and at the same time maintain all essential metabolic activity. In particular, a fuel supply for the brain must be provided for. With this concept in mind, we will next consider how and when to fuel for exercise and recovery. We will also underscore again the important role that honey may play in fueling for exercise and recovery.

Ten Basic Fueling Facts

1. The primary fuel for exercise in humans is glucose, a simple carbohydrate.
2. The greater the intensity of exercise, the greater percentage of glucose burned relative to fat.
3. The most significant energy storehouse for exercise and recovery is the liver glycogen store.
4. Fueling for muscles and liver should be undertaken before, during and after exercise, and with respect to the liver, prior to recovery sleep.
5. Fructose is the sugar specifically selected by the liver to facilitate and regulate glucose uptake.
6. A fructose-based fuel during exercise will increase oxidation and therefore power output during exercise.
7. Optimal fueling of both muscles and liver will reduce production of adrenal stress hormones and protect muscle proteins from degradation.
8. Optimal fueling is as important during training as it is for competition. [*In one sense it is more important, because it is the daily metabolic toll during training that will impact the athlete's health over the period of an athlete's competitive life, both in the short and long term.*]
9. Fats are never a limiting factor during exercise being abundantly available. Any attempt to release extra fats during exercise will be counter-productive and promote long term negative consequences.
10. Proteins may be a significant fuel used during exercise, however good fueling protocols must be followed taking into account the liver. The liver glycogen storehouse is critical.

7 How and When to Fuel for Exercise

Chapter Summary

Fueling for exercise must be primarily concerned with proper liver fueling as the liver is the primary storehouse for brain fuel. Optimum liver fueling protects from muscle protein degradation due to release of adrenal stress hormones when liver stores run low.

There are five critical times for providing fuel to the body in preparation for exercise. They are:

- On rising
- Before exercise
- During exercise
- Post exercise
- Before recovery sleep

The need to include fructose in fuel for exercise is crucial. Fructose regulates glucose uptake into the liver and serves as a substrate for formation of liver glycogen.

"Hepatheletes" are liver-conscious, utilizing proper methods of fueling the liver for exercise.

Honey is a high-octane fuel for exercise.

Several negative health consequences are the result of poor liver fueling in athletes.

This discussion of how and when to fuel for exercise will focus on the role of the liver in fueling the brain (the liver glycogen store is referred to as the liver/brain axis). This is the system that is universally ignored by most trainers and coaches, professional and recreational athletes, and is not covered in most sports' science institutions. Optimum fueling of the liver protects muscle protein from degradation by reducing the production and release of adrenal stress hormones. It is not our intention to write a comprehensive manual on the various types of foods required for any athlete to fuel for any specific exercise. This information is available in a variety of sport manuals, textbooks, popular exercise and sports magazines and other sporting literature. It is our goal, however, to provide the recreational or professional athlete general guidelines for fueling for exercise during the day. Throughout this discussion, the state of the liver glycogen store at critical periods will be underscored.

The Five Critical Times for Fueling

There are five times during a 24-hour day which are critical for proper exercise fueling. These critical times are:

- On rising
- Before exercise
- During exercise
- Post exercise
- Before recovery sleep

On Rising

Mother was right. The day should always begin with a good healthy breakfast. But the reason has to do more with physiology and liver glycogen than it does with following mother's advice. In the early morning hours or upon awakening, the liver requires attention. Glycogen stores are nearly depleted after eight hours of sleep, assuming one retired with a fully stocked liver. The brain, if it has not begun to do so already, is responding to the increasing IGFBP-1 levels from the liver and is correctly sensing that its fuel supply is low.

A healthy drink of *100% fruit juice* easily and rapidly corrects this situation. Notice the emphasis on 100% fruit juice. It is almost tragic to have to point this out, but much of the fruit juice sold in the market today is blended fruit juice sweetened with HFCS. Pure 100% juice of most varieties has just the right amount of fructose and glucose. Adding HFCS does nothing beneficial and only leads to the complications and negative health challenges discussed in Chapter 2.

Most of us are aware of just what a good breakfast consists of, although for a variety of reasons we do not always adhere to this knowledge and follow good practice. Whole grain cereals are excellent with fruits and/or fruit juice or plain yogurt with honey for optimal liver replenishment. Remember it is fructose in combination with glucose from natural sources such as fruit or honey that serves to refuel the liver best. Fructose uptake and fructose-driven glucose uptake into the liver (the Fructose Paradox from Chapter 2) are key elements to keep in mind for this first fuel stop of the day. If you are having a difficult time weaning yourself off of the high calorie, low nutrition breakfast cereals, then at least add a dose of honey for sweetener to provide fructose and glucose in proper combination.

Quality protein in the forms of eggs, low fat cheese, lean meat or even fish may also be eaten at this time. If time is at a premium, some 300-500 milliliters (about 10-16 ounces) of a quality 100% fruit drink will provide the correct fructose/glucose balance to optimize liver uptake.

If exercise, such as an early morning run is on your agenda, you should not initiate this activity without fueling. Unfortunately exercising without fueling is a common practice in the recreational and professional athletic community, especially among those hoping to burn extra fat. *This will not and cannot happen.* Exercise will prompt the release of adrenal hormones, which will in turn mobilize extra fats. These fats will not be oxidized. They will cycle around the circulatory system until the exercise is over, and most will simply be returned to fat stores in the adipose tissue.

The best fueling advice if exercising in the morning is to allow at least 90 minutes after a light breakfast before beginning your routine to allow for digestion and storage of foods. Then about 30 minutes before exercise have a small fruit snack or some fruit with honey. This will best prepare the athlete for a morning exercise session.

One additional important point should be raised here. Athletes will sometimes refer to feeling "like superman" in the morning, thus concluding that they have no requirement for fueling prior to exercise. This would be a very foolish enterprise. Even when the liver was optimally fueled prior to bed, it would still be depleted on rising. For any athlete who retired to bed with low liver glycogen, and entered a state of adrenal stress overnight, the blood glucose concentration may be elevated in the early morning.

This phenomenon, known as the **"Dawn Phenomenon"** (described on p. 70), results from the activity of cortisol and adrenaline which mobilize energy stores in order to create new glucose from degraded protein. It is a well recognized danger for diabetics who may show a **falsely** elevated level of blood glucose, and misjudge their insulin dosage requirements. Trained athletes have enhanced adrenal efficiency. Therefore this phenomenon may occur in such athletes, giving a very false impression of the liver glycogen status. An early morning exercise training session undertaken in that circumstance would promote a tide of additional adrenal hormone release. The benefit of the exercise session would be cancelled out with extra protein losses.

Before Exercise

The timing of fueling prior to exercise is profoundly related to the timing of the previous meal. Optimally, it is best to eat around three hours before exercise to allow time for digestion and storage of fuels. A small snack may be eaten around 90 minutes before beginning an exercise protocol, some cereal with fruit or fruit with honey. Then it is a good idea to top off the liver with fruit juice or honey 15 to 30 minutes before a race or a workout. This last fueling protocol takes into account liver depletion during the last hour or so before the workout, something most fueling manuals ignore. Keep in mind that the brain monitors fuel stores and rates of depletion of blood glucose from the hypothalamus. This region of the brain is located in the limbic system, the unconscious part of the brain. This part of the brain operates independently of the cortex, our higher level "thinking" region of the brain.

Our hunter-gatherer ancestors would set out in the morning food seeking, cognizant of the constant danger from predators. They were physiologically built to react to such threats by activating the "fight or flight" physiology. However, in such circumstances, the brain is faced with a difficult dilemma. How much fuel does it allow contracting muscles to extract from the circulation and how much will be retained for its own use?

In the event of a good energy status liver glycogen indication, the brain may allow for increased power output, thus increasing the potential for survival from a predator threat. This increased power output must be balanced by the need to conserve the fuel supply for the brain. The result is absolutely dependent on the liver energy status at any given time, as the liver is the only store supplying glucose both to the brain and contracting muscles. All other metabolic considerations will become secondary to this at such critical times. The hypothalamus will be monitoring this question every nanosecond during the period of threat and will decide the response, independent of the thinking processes of the subject involved.

A race is not physiologically different. The competing athlete may know in his/her conscious mind that a 100 meter race will come to an end in about ten seconds. The hypothalamus will make its fuel calculations based on a worst case scenario - that of a continuing chase - and will allow fuel utilization and therefore power output according to fuel and energy status. This status will always be based above all other fuel stores on liver energy status or liver glycogen plenitude. The athlete is running for glory and a medal, the hypothalamus is insuring its own survival. The predator may be running for its lunch, the human subject is running for his/her life. The liver glycogen status will determine the outcome.

For this reason all exercise poses a threat to the brain. The brain must constantly legislate between fuel supply to contracting muscles and preserving its own metabolic life. This is precisely why the adrenal hormones create such confusion in sport literature where glucose uptake into contracting muscles during such "fight or flight" episodes is the only consideration. Adrenal hormones are actually released to protect fuel supply to the brain. **They are neuro-protective hormones.** Therefore, if your race lasts ten seconds or over ten hours, liver plenitude must be factored into your fueling protocols, before, during, and after exercise, as well as during recovery.

During Exercise

Fueling during exercise and or participation in sports is obviously going to be somewhat dependent on the sport undertaken. Clearly it is possible to fuel during endurance exercise on a bike as you can easily carry fuel with you, but other protocols such as swimming, running, and skiing present the athlete with challenges. Regardless of the sport, the key is to fuel to whatever maximum when possible.

Until recent years most sport energy drinks were based on glucose and or glucose polymers, which are metabolized rapidly into glucose. Fructose was panned in the literature for several reasons. In the concentrations initially used in studies, fructose caused gut distress. These concentrations were actually much higher than what is found in natural foods. The fructose found in foods is most always balanced with glucose. Furthermore, because muscle cells did not take up fructose during exercise, it was not considered as effective for muscle fueling as glucose.

This view was in line with the general perspective of "liver blindness" which was and remains prevalent in sports. In recent years, however there has been an increased interest in fructose as a fuel. Sport or exercise fuels can now be found which contain fructose along with glucose and/or glucose polymers (chains of repeated glucose units).

With any moderate intensity exercise protocol the optimum is to rehydrate up to 1 liter per hour and to include in this around 60 grams of carbohydrate. This carbohydrate should include about 20% glucose, 20% fructose and 60% of maltodextrins. In longer endurance protocols energy bars and gels may be used as well as sport drinks, again keeping firmly in mind that fructose is vital, so that glucose uptake into liver is optimized.

There is one physiological truth, one unsung secret of exercise physiology that needs to be underscored and preached to every sporting youth or adult, every recreational or professional athlete, every coach and sport physiologist. It is this:

Glucokinase must be unlocked from the liver cell and available to allow for glucose uptake by the liver during exercise. Exercise inhibits glucokinase release, but fructose will release this enzyme. Fueling during exercise with fructose and glucose in a balanced ratio facilitates glucose uptake into the liver and promotes glycogen formation. The result is improved power output, improved mental acuity, improved psychology and improved recovery. And with improved recovery comes the added bonus of improved overall health.

Post Exercise Refueling

There are some important considerations to keep in mind in the post-exercise period. The key to refueling in the post-exercise period is to refuel as quickly as possible after exercise. This not only optimizes replenishment of fuel stores, in particular muscle glycogen, but also readies the body for optimum recovery physiology. Many coaches will recommend a protein supplement immediately after exercise and this is perfectly in order. In the immediate post-exercise period usually lasting about two hours, uptake of protein is optimized. It makes good sense to take advantage of this. Also the replenishment of muscle glycogen is improved when carbohydrates are ingested during this period along with protein.

The post-exercise replenishment of muscle glycogen may also be achieved with carbohydrate drinks or food. Suitable foods are whole grain breads, pasta, rice and potatoes - these foods are glucose based and the metabolic environment at this period is optimal for muscle replenishment.

During exercise, contracting muscles extract glucose from the circulation with great efficiency. This may seem contradictory because insulin is suppressed during exercise and muscle cells normally require insulin signaling to effect this uptake. However contracting muscles extract glucose from the circulation by developing a system independent of insulin known as *exercise induced muscle uptake of glucose.*[149] As each muscle cell contracts, the glucose transporters are driven to the cell wall allowing for rapid glucose uptake - a process normally requiring insulin.

This system, independent of and complementary to insulin, remains in place for up to 48 hours in the post-exercise period and this ensures good muscle glycogen replenishment. Muscle cells will extract up to 90% of available glucose during this period. In addition to this exercise induced mechanism, insulin will also be released in response to carbohydrate intake, and this will be additive to the exercise induced mechanism.[150]

The post-exercise refueling period must also give attention to replenishing the liver glycogen stores. This will occur if one includes some fructose containing foods, such as fruits and vegetables or honey, which ensure liver uptake of glucose. However, any liver glycogen formed will be quickly released from the liver in this period to provide glucose for depleted muscle tissue as referred to above. Therefore it is also recommended to do some selective refueling of the liver in the post-exercise period prior to bed time when recovery physiology is the key metabolic consideration.

Before Recovery Sleep

Some sport and exercise fueling literature and manuals will suggest a snack before bed, but fail to offer any explanation as to why this may be significant, or give consideration to the importance of fueling the liver glycogen store. This is entirely in keeping with the generalized "liver blindness" prevalent in modern sport mentioned earlier.

The absolute overriding consideration during this critical time for fueling is the liver glycogen status. If we assume that the post-exercise refueling from foods, beverages and/or supplements is adequate to replenish muscle glycogen storage, and we have included protein and fats to provide the building materials necessary for repair and reconstruction of tissues, then the last and vital consideration is that of selective replenishment of the liver glycogen store. An adequate liver glycogen store is foundational to provide the optimal metabolic environment for recovery physiology during sleep.

Honey as Fuel for Recovery Sleep

Honey is the best possible food for this purpose. Not only does honey provide the correct balance of fructose to glucose, but it will optimally and selectively refuel the liver, without a significant digestive burden during recovery sleep. This is an important consideration as digestion is a metabolically expensive and energy demanding series of physiologic processes. The amount of honey necessary prior to bed time will vary according to body size and the status of liver glycogen stores just before sleep. Typically, one or two tablespoons would provide optimum fuel to ensure adequate liver glycogen during recovery sleep. When adequate liver glycogen stores are available during sleep, fat burning will be optimized during that time.

Honey as a Fuel for Exercise

If you were researching fuels to find which fuel would be most suitable for your sport or exercise regime it would seem reasonable to look at the fuels used by the world's most successful athletes. You would give consideration to the type of exercise and the physical effort required in terms of power output and endurance and make fuel selection accordingly.

Many studies have been performed on exercise metabolism using animal models, most often rats and mice, and we are able to learn much from this approach. These comparative animal studies have yielded up much valuable information on metabolic pathways, enzyme dynamics and hormones that respond to alterations in fuel availability, both during exercise and the post-exercise refueling period.

Exercise metabolism studies using mammals of various types offer excellent comparisons to humans, but other animal orders such as insects have been less studied. Surprisingly these may also yield important insights. Certainly insects perform feats of power output and endurance that humans may only dream of.

Many entomologists regard the humble honeybee as one example of supreme athletic prowess for several good reasons. Consider the speed and distances that honeybees travel for instance. A honeybee may achieve airborne speeds of up to 10 mph and travel for up to 10 miles. These are amazing speed and endurance stats for an insect weighing in at less than 0.5 grams. On an equivalent weight to speed basis, a 75 kilo human could reach a speed of nearly 1.5 million miles per hour, an absurd yet illustrative example.

What is it about the honeybee that allows it to achieve such levels of performance output even to the extent that it may seem to defy the laws of exercise metabolism and even physics? One famous French entomologist actually claimed that bee flight was not possible in spite of observed reality.

There is one aspect of honeybee physiology that may prove significant in contrast to humans. Honeybees have what we can refer to as an open fuel storage and circulation system. Humans have what is in effect a closed or segmented fuel storage system. Contracting muscles utilize intracellular muscle glycogen stores and may also access liver glycogen stores during exercise. Depletion of the liver glycogen store places the brain at risk of fuel shortages, forcing it to release adrenal stress hormones to insure adequate fuel supply for brain functioning.

Honeybees have no such challenge. The honeybee brain and its contracting wing muscles have open access to the same fuel store at all times. In the unlikely event that a bee runs short of fuel, both its brain and muscles will run out at the precisely the same moment.

In exercising humans, the brain must be fueled exclusively from the liver glycogen store while contracting muscles may be fueled from both muscle glycogen and liver glycogen. An early warning fuel detection system is essential so that the liver may warn the brain of an impending fuel shortage. Beginning with the onset of exercise and throughout the exercise duration, the liver signals the brain via IGFBP-1 when its fuel store is running low. As IGFBP-1 is released, it binds and inhibits IGF-1. As discussed in Chapter 7, IGF-1 is a very powerful insulin-like signaling protein that drives glucose into muscles. When IGF-1 is bound and inhibited by IGFBP-1, less glucose is taken in by contracting muscles, thus keeping more glucose in circulation. However, the tradeoff is that less glucose oxidation takes place within muscle cells at a significant reduction in power output.

This important physiological difference between exercising honeybees and humans may not explain the vast differential in athletic efficiency. However if we look at fueling protocols we may detect just why these differences exist. Honeybees use two fuels in flight, nectar and honey. When a honeybee leaves the hive to forage for nectar and pollen, it fuels up on honey, but in the course of foraging, the honey will gradually be replaced by nectar. Although honey is derived from nectar and transformed into a miraculous fuel by the honeybee, nectar and honey are not the same. Nectar is composed primarily of sucrose while honey is composed of nearly equal quantities of free fructose and free glucose. This difference may account for some of the variation in fuel dynamics.

The key to the amazing flight dynamics of honeybees may be provided by looking at the metabolism of these two fuels. Studies have previously shown that honey is an excellent fuel in endurance exercise providing stable blood glucose control.[151] However, these studies were of limited value as they made no direct comparison of honey to sucrose, the nearest compositional equivalent. Furthermore, the authors made no attempt to examine or explain the metabolic dynamics of honey in exercise and recovery.

Honey, as you are now well aware, is a nearly one-to-one ratio of fructose to glucose. The key is that the sugars exist as free molecules. Sucrose has an exact one-to-one ratio of glucose to fructose but the sugars are bound as a double sugar (disaccharide) requiring separation by enzyme hydrolysis in the gut, before absorption. The free fructose from honey is absorbed much more rapidly than is glucose. Here we have the first gluco-regulatory role for fructose in so far as fructose will reach the liver first and unlock glucokinase from the liver cell nuclei, allowing for the uptake of glucose into the liver and its conversion to glycogen. In combination with protein, honey is an excellent post-exercise food for recovery.

The Role of Fructose in Exercise Fueling

After decades of being ignored or panned in sports physiology literature, fructose is emerging as one of the most significant fuels in human exercise metabolism. The reasons that fructose was overlooked are several. Early studies on fructose used it in high concentrations, much higher than those found in nature or natural foods. High fructose concentrations typically led to gastric distress.[152] Other references on exercise fueling claimed that because fructose would not be taken up by muscles and used to form muscle glycogen, it could not be used by contracting muscles and thus was of little use as an exercise fuel.

It is precisely because this occurs that fructose is so important. Fructose serves as a substrate for formation of liver glycogen and more than that, it regulates glucose uptake into the liver. The liver fuel store, is as we have pointed out, the key fuel depot in human exercise metabolism.

Military Myopia

This secret truth behind unlocking glucokinase from the liver cell nuclei is especially applicable in the prevention of a particular type of military myopia. Every young person in the military is required to be physically fit, and is personally responsible to ensure this is the case. Maximum fitness above all means the ability for fast neural processing and mental acuity in situations of danger.

When we examine the field rations provided as fuel for this optimum fitness, a number of concerns are raised. Frequently, these rations are supplied with maximum energy density as the main imperative. But energy density in the form of fats and chocolate is not optimal for neural processing. Field rations are not supplied with the type of fructose based foods that may optimize these metabolic requirements.

Military fitness necessary for action and life protection requires that decisions be made acutely and rapidly. Foods and fuels should provide for optimal liver/brain axis fueling. It seems this is a subject to which the military culinary and food requisition experts should pay particular attention.

In recent years, researchers at Birmingham University in England, have taken up the study of fructose in exercise and come to some outstanding conclusions. One particular study, by Jeukendrup and his team, published in 2005 in the Journal of Applied Physiology is of relevant significance.[153]

Eight well-trained subjects exercised three times at 58% maximum oxygen consumption, while ingesting either a glucose drink or a glucose/fructose drink in a ratio of 2:1. Both fuels were delivered at concentrations of 9%. The study was seeking to establish if consumption of these drinks could maintain carbohydrate oxidation during the latter stages of a five hour exercise protocol, and if there would be increased oxidation of ingested (exogenous) carbohydrate.

What they found was quite dramatic. The results showed increased rates of carbohydrate oxidation in the glucose/fructose group significantly above that of the glucose only group, late in exercise. They also found better endurance as indicated by improvements in maintaining cadence (measured by revolutions per minute) in the fructose containing fuel group, and in reduced perceived rates of exertion (RPE).

Although the study by Jeukendrup and associates did not look directly at a psychological effect of fructose fueling, this subjective finding deserves additional investigation. They did find significant reductions in "perception of gastric volume" in the fructose group, suggesting improved gastric emptying and improved water absorption. Again these are potent findings, not only in terms of performance but in the absorption and usage of fuels during exercise and in improved hydration.

The rate of appearance of glucose did not match the rate of oxidation. This suggests that some other form of fuel sourced from available glucose was being oxidized. The authors suggested that this may be lactate (a 3-carbon fragment of glucose or fructose). It is known that fructose metabolism may also increase lactate levels. Lactate was observed to rise significantly in this study. Lactate may be taken up and oxidized by contracting muscles. Fructose is an excellent molecule for formation of trioses - 3-carbon fragments - suggesting the release of lactate from liver. The uptake and utilization of lactate would not compete with glucose uptake into muscle cells.

That lactate may now be regarded as a significant exercise fuel may be viewed as a benefit from including fructose in one's exercise fueling regimen. [154] In other words, the release of lactate from the liver during exercise may provide another source of energy to contracting muscles from the glucose/ fructose pool. The resultant increased oxidation of carbohydrate fuel equates to increased power output.

Not unexpectedly, the authors did not refer to the significance of the formation of liver glycogen during the exercise protocol. If during the protocol, liver glycogen was being formed, as a result of fructose liver uptake, and the liberation of glucokinase - the liver glucose enzyme - we now would have our presumed mechanism for improved glucose oxidation from ingested glucose.

Another year long animal study from New Zealand by Starkey, Chepulis and their associates, showed that honey improved memory and reduced anxiety in rats, as compared to sucrose, suggesting improved glucose metabolism in neural cells.[155]

These findings are in line with the ideas postulated in **The Hibernation Diet**, that fructose containing fuels are superior to sucrose or glucose alone. These results suggest that fructose will play a potent role in neural processing during endurance exercise, a finding we have heard many times from individual athletes.

The Role of IGFBP-1 Revisited

Formation of new liver glycogen during exercise will *reduce* the release of IGFBP-1. This in turn will free up IGF-1 and allow glucose transport into contracting muscles, thus improving glucose oxidation and therefore power output. The use of a glucose/fructose energy drink during endurance exercise, as opposed to pure glucose, therefore will positively improve a range of exercise parameters including power output in the later stages of prolonged exercise.

By optimally fueling the liver, an athlete will optimally fuel contracting muscles. To put it another way: ***Powering the liver powers muscles!***

While no available exercise fueling studies compare honey directly to sucrose, a number of studies do compare honey to sucrose from various other perspectives, such as blood glucose and triglyceride levels. Honey always comes out favorably in such studies.[156] These studies may be explained by the improved glucose disposal and metabolism of glucose from honey, compared to glucose obtained from sucrose.

What are the constituent differences between sucrose and honey, and in what way may these differences affect the metabolic outcome? Honey is laden with glucose metabolizing principles, vitamins, amino acids, minerals, bioflavonoids, organic acid volatiles, and other ingredients, such as nitric oxide and hydrogen peroxide. These act at low levels to promote insulin signaling, in different signaling pathways, and therefore act to improve glucose uptake, disposal and oxidation in muscle cells. These may explain many of the metabolic benefits of honey, as compared to all other refined sugars and carbohydrates. Since exercise is a particular form of heightened metabolic activity that places the requirement for fuel homeostasis above all other metabolic parameters, we may have our explanation why honey is such a potent metabolic exercise fuel.

Although there are no available studies comparing honey to sucrose in human exercise, there is one that compares nectar and honey to sucrose as a fuel powering flight in parasitoid wasps.[157] Not surprisingly honey comes out ahead of sucrose in improving flight dynamics. This is significant. The metabolic principles in honey drive forward glucose metabolism by insulin activism, and may be expected to improve glucose disposal both at rest and during exercise. Any improvement in glucose metabolism in contracting muscle cells during exercise will improve exercise dynamics, and this result will be in addition to the metabolic benefits of fructose discussed above.

The "Hepathelete" is an Informed, Liver-conscious Athlete

Searching for a hepathlon, may get one directed to an athletic event known as the heptathlon, a seven event track and field contest that is included in the Olympics. An athlete who competes in this grueling event is known as a heptathlete, the name deriving from the Greek hepta (seven) and athlon (contest). As far as we know there is no event known as the hepathlon. However, it may be instructive to describe an informed athlete as a hepathlete.

What is a hepathlete, and in what way would such an athlete differ from other athletes?

A hepathlete is:
- A liver conscious athlete (from *hepatikos*, Greek: of the liver)
- An athlete who is acutely aware that in human metabolism and physiology, the liver is the significant fuel store both during exercise and during recovery
- Conscious of the role of liver glycogen and its relation to brain metabolism, insofar as the liver is the only store that releases glucose to the circulation, a function vital for maintaining fuel supply to the brain during exercise
- An athlete who is aware of when and by what means the liver may be optimally fueled before, during, after exercise and prior to recovery during the night fast
- Aware of the central role of fructose in human metabolism, of how it is taken up by the liver cell and converted to glucose and then stored as liver glycogen if blood glucose is stable, or released to the circulation, if required, when blood glucose is falling
- Aware of the critical role of fructose in liberating the liver glucose enzyme, glucokinase from the liver cell, and therefore of its role in regulating glucose uptake into the liver at critical times, again during exercise and during recovery
- Aware of the critical 1:1 ratio of fructose to glucose - the optimum ratio that allows fructose regulation of glucose uptake into the liver - and of the foods that provide this ideal ratio, fruits and honey
- Aware of the role of liver glycogen during exercise, how it maintains fuel supply to the brain, how it regulates power output by modulating release of IGFBP-1, the central fuel gauge in human exercise metabolism, and how improving liver glycogen plenitude during exercise with a fructose based fuel in the correct percentage will reduce the release of IGFBP-1, free up IGF-1, improve glucose uptake into contracting muscles, increase glucose oxidation, and therefore increase power output

Api-Athlete

An api-athlete ("api" is a prefix taken from the Latin word apis, meaning bee) may be described as an athlete who utilizes honey much as bees do as a potent fuel for exercise. The api-athlete also recognizes that honey is the ideal food for replenishing the liver glycogen store both prior to exercise and prior to recovery sleep.

We seek to encourage exercise physiologists and sports scientists to take up the study of honey and compare its benefits with other exercise fuels in equivalent sugar ratios. When sport science faculties look at various exercise fuels, a variety of carbohydrates combined in differing ratios should be considered. As the liver becomes more and more a focus of these studies, new information will accrue, and new paradigms will be established about the relationship between central (or hepatic) and peripheral (or muscle) metabolism.

We expect honey to feature increasingly in these studies, not simply because it contains the optimum ratio of free sugars, but because each dose of honey is blessed with a potent army of glucose metabolizing principles. Such principles will optimize glucose metabolism in contracting muscles with significant impact on glucose oxidation and power output.

High Octane Honey

We already know what many of these principles are - vanadium, chromium, bioflavonoids, nitric oxide, hydrogen peroxide and so on - and there may be others that are not yet discovered. What we do know is that a flying honeybee may reach levels of fuel oxidation and power output undreamed of in human metabolism. We know that of the two fuels used by honeybees, nectar and honey, honey is a higher octane fuel, insofar as it is lower in water concentration than is nectar and contains the right balance of fructose and sucrose.

Therefore, what is the highest octane natural fuel available to humans during exercise and sport? To pose the question is to answer it.

Honey is the highest octane natural fuel available to humans, for exercise and sport and with the added dividend, for recovery!

The Psychology and Power of Honey and Liver Fueling

Whenever athletes engage in optimal liver fueling prior to and during exercise a powerful psychological bonus is expressed. Although this benefit may be expected to occur during endurance workouts when the liver would be depleted, this also occurs during short periods of anaerobic workouts lasting as little as ten seconds. During these protocols there is no possibility that the liver could deplete to any significant extent, but the psychological benefit of optimal liver fueling is expressed by such athletes, in exactly the same terms as that of endurance athletes.

Frequently athletes will express that they "felt strong," "had a clear head," "had no negative thoughts," "felt great," "had a very positive race." Any athlete who is well prepared physically and psychologically prior to an event should end with a sense of optimism and clear-headedness (endorphine production from exercise not withstanding). This optimism would originate from the conscious part of the brain (the cortex) and would not necessarily be mirrored by input from the hypothalmus, the region associated with monitoring fuel availability (as described in Chapter 5). But why would there be such a potent psychological impact from optimal liver fueling with short exercise protocols that would not significantly deplete the liver?

To answer this, we need to briefly explore what connections there may be between optimal liver fueling and one's psychological state. Most of us are aware that when we are hungry and eat something enjoyable, there is an immediate feeling of relief combined with a surge of apparent energy. This surge cannot be due to new energy reserves being ready to fuel activity because of the time lag between ingestion, digestion, storage and availability. It is the sensitivity and rapidity of response of the hormones of the hypothalmus and the SCN (see pages 58, 59) that monitor and regulate energy availability and expenditure that give indications of actual energy state well ahead of cortical awareness. The conscious portion of the brain receives indications of an energy surge before any reserves are actually available.

The reverse senario is also true as the view from the hypothalmus is always based on liver glycogen status. When liver glycogen is low, power output will, of, necessity be reduced. The monitoring and regulatory function of the hyothalamus will run ahead of the athlete's actual fuel demand and make this adjustment in advance of such a fuel shortage. Thus the athlete who fails to prime the liver before an exercise protocol will suffer from a kind of hypothalamic pesimissim, a strategy that will induce fatigue even before fuel reserves are exhausted.

Proper fueling preparation by paying attention to liver glycogen stores allows the hypothalamus some degree of "relaxation" in terms of anticipated energy release. This in turn allows optimistic cortical sensations. This psychological bonus, deriving from optimal liver fueling, is exactly what these athletes have experienced and described.

This effect is probably also related to sublingual (under the tongue) absorption of certain fuels. Sublingual rate of absorption occurs immediately at a rate much more rapid than from the gut. Thus if an athlete takes a sip of a liver fueling drink in the last seconds before an event and retains some in the mouth during the last seconds prior to the gun he would experience a slightly delayed surge of positivism from his cortex.

A remarkable study completed in 2004 provides confirmation of this. A bicycling team got the idea of studying the effect of carbohydrates in mouthwash as a boost to performance. Previous studies had shown no beneficial effect from glucose infusions (as opposed to an oral drink) on performance in a simulated 40k time trial . The carbohydrate rinse was used regularly during a one hour cycling time trial. Performance times were significantly faster in the carbohydrate trial group compared with those given a placebo - an average of 59.57 minutes compared with 61.37 minutes - representing a 2.9% improvement. Power output with the carbohydrate rinse was correspondingly higher in the trial group measured at 259 watts compared with 252 watts for those given the placebo. These results were observed even though the athletes rinsed their mouths with the carbohydrate drink and then ejected it. The authors speculated that oral receptors in the mouth would register the incoming fuel. They did not consider sublingual absorption as providing instantaneous direct input via the cerebral circulation.

Clearly there was some physiological effect on output derived from the oral ingestion of fuel as opposed to infusion. "These results suggest," they explain, "that oral carbohydrate may exert its effects during high-intensity exercise through a central action, improving motor drive or motivation, mediated by receptors in the mouth or GI tract."[158] This psychological enhancement in anticipation of any actual physiologic benefit is exactly what we experience when we eat something we enjoy, like chocolate.

The first positive indication that optimal liver fuelling would have potential for improving short exercise protocols came to the attention of the authors in early August 2004. A young middle distance athlete was given a sample of our honey-based liver fuel along with a suggestion that he try it out. Soon after, he responded to us in an email to tell us that the effect on his training physiology was profound, taking minutes off his 3 x 2 mile protocol with the added factor of a vast improvement in his mental state.

He again emailed a few days later to say he was taking seconds off his 300 meter repititions and in the final sprint took 1.1 seconds off his time (from 39.8 to 38.7). His appended comments included words like "felt fantastic," "strong," and "great."

At that time we suspected that power output during such short protocols might have been inhibited relative to the glycogen status of the liver. We now know that the pathway by which energy expenditure is reduced involves IGFBP-1 inhibition of IGF-1 which results in reduced delivery of glucose into muscle (see pp. 86-89). Benjamin Libet and his work with the cycling team cited above discovered that unconscious processing in the hypothalamus occurs some 500 millieseconds ahead of cortical recognition. Any athlete may take advantage of this aspect of physiology by ingesting a fructose based fuel in the seconds prior to engaging in a power protocol. The anticipation of incoming fuel will be flashed to the cortex via sublingual uptake thus combining the impact of a positive psychological state with power released via inhibition of IGFBP-1.

We have herein shown that liver glycogen status is the most significant factor affecting both power output and psychology during any exercise protocol. The length of the protocol is not relevant. Many top athletes spend a great deal of money on hiring sport psychologists. They could more easily improve their mental and psycological state before a race by becoming liver conscious and taking advantage of the power of honey.

A rookie sprint car race driver from north central Kansas, Nate Brown, a points leader among a field of 32 other drivers, many with 10 or more years of experience, described both the psychological and physiological benefit beautifully: "The one thing that makes the biggest impact on my race is taking a honey stix (a plastic straw containing honey) about 5 minutes before each race. About that time, I ususally get nervous and shaky, so much so that I cannot hold my hands still. After the honey stix I am very quickly calmed down. And my mind is cleared!"

McArdle's Disease, a Useful Model for Liver Blindness in Sports Physiology

Brian McArdle, was the second son of Andrew McArdle, who at the time was parliamentary correspondent for The Scotsman. After studying medicine, he took a post in Guy's Hospital in London. He spent the years during World War II studying the effect of heat and cold on troops, methods for the prevention of trench foot, and how to prevent sea-sickness. Knowing that troops had to be combat ready from the moment they landed, he pioneered the use of hyoscine for sea-sickness. This drug was administered to the troops embarking for the D-Day landings and in spite of rough sea conditions, the majority did not experience this malady on the cross-Channel passage. Dr. McArdle discovery was a major contribution to the success of the Normandy landings.

It is for another reason, however, that Dr. McArdle is still known and celebrated in medicine. In 1951 he described a young man with a lifelong history of exercise-induced muscle pain and stiffness, symptoms that previous physicians had dismissed as hysterical. On examination he noted that, unlike ordinary cramps, those experienced by the patient were not accompanied by altered electrical activity and that his venous blood lactate levels did not increase with anaerobic exercise. McArdle noted that these were the same findings that occur in muscle tissue exposed to high levels of iodoacetate, a substance that blocks the metabolism of glycogen into glucose and prevents the formation of lactic acid. McArdle reasoned that the absence of lactic acid formation during exercise was indicating a defect in muscle glucose availability, and therefore suggestive of impaired muscle glycogen breakdown.

His discovery became the first detailed description of metabolic muscle myopathy. Dr. McArdle correctly concluded that the patient had a disorder of glycogen breakdown specifically affecting contracting skeletal muscle. A few years later in 1959, the specific enzyme (muscle phosphorylase or myophosphorylase) deficiency responsible for the patient's symptoms was identified and named by W. F. H. M. Mommaerts.[159]

McArdle's disease is now well recognized as the most common of a number of glycogen storage diseases. It is known as glycogen storage disease type V (GSD-V) and is caused by a genetic deficiency of the myophosphorylase enzyme. This enzyme is necessary to break down glycogen (stored glucose) in muscle tissue during exercise and allows stored glucose to be made available to provide the energy to power muscle contractions. Glucose for powering muscle contractions comes from two different sources, muscle glycogen and blood (therefore liver) glucose, extracted from the circulation during exercise.

In recent years the authors met with a McArdle's patient, Brian Murphy. Brian is a keen recreational exerciser who refused to be defined or limited by his condition. He continued in his attempts at exercising even though this is a singularly difficult achievement for one with McArdle's disease. As exercise is undertaken, contracting muscles have no access to muscle glycogen stores. The only source of glucose must therefore be from blood and liver glycogen stores.

This results in immediate activation of metabolic stress, because the rapid extraction of glucose from the circulation depletes liver glucose and places the brain at metabolic risk. In other words the metabolic response to loss of liver glycogen during exercise, is doubly accelerated in McArdle's patients, and the predictable result is enhanced metabolic stress with increased levels of cortisol and adrenaline being produced. Secondarily there is increased risk of all the adrenal stress-driven diseases that we characterize as the metabolic syndrome.

McArdle's Disease and Liver Glycogen

It was clear to the authors that if Brian were to selectively refuel the liver before and during exercise, he may reduce the level of adrenal activation, and therefore would theoretically reduce the loss of muscle protein. As it turns out, he was already doing exactly that to some extent by consuming quantities of preserved fruits in syrup. Though this was not the best source of natural fructose, it was certainly a source of liver fuel for Brian. He had arrived at a liver fueling strategy empirically and was already having some success.

We suggested a modification to Brian's conscious liver fueling strategy using a fructose (honey-based) formula prior to and during exercise. We also suggested that he consume honey prior to bedtime as a liver replenishment, one that would optimize recovery physiology and facilitate the building of new lean muscle tissue.

The results over some months were dramatic. Brian's exercise capacity increased, and he experienced measurable gains in lean muscle mass along with loss of adipose tissue. When he presented these results to his clinicians, he was surprised that the results of his liver fueling strategy provoked little interest.

This example serves to illustrate the striking parallel between McArdle's patients and any athlete undertaking intense training without adequate liver fueling. In one, the fuel store is blocked and unavailable and in the other, the fuel system is low and running on reserve. The metabolic response to both conditions is the activation of adrenal stress hormones and the degradation of muscle protein to provide backup and replenishment fuel for low liver glycogen stores. However, in McArdles's patients intense exercise may lead to more severe muscle breakdown or rhabdomyolitis, a condition of acute muscle destruction with leakage of cellular toxins into the blood stream and the production of dark urine.

Many an athlete will claim that there is no requirement for fueling during short periods of exercise lasting up to 60 minutes. This does not take into account the metabolic fuel requirements of the brain. During any exercise protocol, liver glycogen status is constantly monitored with IGFBP-1 being released when glycogen stores run low. Activation of metabolic stress to insure adequate glucose for the brain occurs at the instant the liver begins to release this warning signal.

Every athlete should be made aware of the nature of McArdle's disease as it provides a sobering look at what can occur during acute metabolic stress. Dealing with McArdle's disease provides all athletes with a model for combating "liver blindness," a condition universal in modern sport. Proper liver fueling is essential for the prevention of metabolic stress.

Muscle Loss and Motor Neuron Disease in Professional Athletes

In situations where athletes overtrain or fail to fuel the liver optimally (this is common situation in both professional and recreational sports), protein metabolism will increase, muscle protein is degraded to produce glucose and muscle cell function compromised. A possible factor that links loss of muscle cell function to motor neuron disease (MND, also known as ALS or Lou Gehrig's disease in the U.S. after the baseball legend who was diagnosed with it in 1939), a disease with increased incidence among athletes, was pointed out to the authors in a personal communication from a Scottish farmer, Tom Stockdale, whose interest in physiology led him to the following profound observation.

Arginine, an amino acid which is considered "conditionally essential" (meaning that it must be supplied exogenously to specific populations that do not synthesize it in adequate amounts) is required to make guanosine monophosphate (GMP), a nucleotide that serves as a gatekeeper for calcium regulation in motor neurons. Arginine can be synthesized from other amino acids in the body. Failure to make or maintain adequate levels of arginine would result in failure to make GMP. The motor neuron end plate, under the regulatory control of GMP, releases calcium into the muscle cell, causing it to contract. Calcium is then pumped out of the cell, allowing for another round of contraction. If GMP is not formed, the cell may fail to excrete calcium and will die. Chronic muscle protein degradation could be responsible for this lack of GMP. Additional studies must be conducted to confirm this hypothesis.

There is now increasing recognition that professional athletes may be at greater risk for MND and that athletic participation itself may be a risk factor for several disease states. A recent investigation was prompted in Italy when it was learned that Italian soccer players had five times the number of cases of MND than the national average. Adriano Chio and his team at Turin University researched the medical records of 7000 professional footballers for MND or ALS.[160] The predicted disease incidence of MND in that number of young men should have been 0.8. In stead the number was five. They also found the average age of onset was 41 years of age, some 20 years earlier than the expected norm.

Clusters of cases have been reported in American football, but until now no large-scale studies have found any clear link between American football and ALS. The MND Society in the United Kingdom has confirmed their concerns about this risk. The aggressive loss of muscle protein during exercise training when fueling protocols are not optimal, combined with chronic increased metabolic stress over a ten to twenty year period in the lives of all young athletes, may be factors underlying some genetic propensity for MND/ALS. It is likely that this may be the case for many professional athletes in many sports.

Additional Benefits of Arginine

Though not related to the above discussion of the possible association of arginine deficiencies with MND, it should be noted that this particular amino acid has important roles to play within the body with regard to cell division, wound healing, ammonia removal from the body and control and release of certain hormones.

Arginine is known to be associated with several additional functions in the body. Reports following the oral ingestion of L-arginine indicate that it may provide the following possible benefits:

- Serves as a precursor for the synthesis of Nitric Oxide (NO)
- Stimulates the release of the most important anti-aging hormone in the body, growth hormone
- Improves immune function
- Reduces healing time of injuries (particularly bone)
- Reduces risk of heart disease
- Increases muscle mass
- Reduces adipose tissue body fat
- Helps improve insulin sensitivity
- Helps decrease blood pressure
- Alleviates male infertility, improving sperm production and motility
- Increases circulation throughout the body, including the sex organs.[161]

The importance of proper fueling during training and competition is again underscored. Strategies that fuel the liver before, during and post-exercise must be directed at securing and maintaining liver glycogen stores and protecting against protein catabolism. To disregard this critical fact places the athlete at risk of a host of metabolic conditions that directly result from protein loss due to metabolic stress.

Auto-cannibalism and Liver Blindness in Athletics

Recycling of muscle proteins and conversion to glucose in the liver (with loss of nitrogen), is a normal aspect of our daily metabolism. This always takes place to some extent over the 24 hour cycle and certainly during exercise. Muscle proteins are vital to all exercise protocols. Every athlete must be aware of how to minimize muscle loss. Every athlete, at every level and of all ages, must become liver conscious - that is knowledgeable of how to fuel the liver optimally before, during, after exercise, and prior to the night fast.

Degradation of muscle protein is directly related to liver glycogen status. The state of recurrent depleted liver glycogen results in excess and unnecessary catabolism of muscle proteins by "liver blind" athletes. We characterize this as a form of auto-cannibalism.

The popular notion that somehow athletic performance and good health are synonymous is coming under increasing scrutiny. The effects of fueling deficiencies during training, associated poor performance and long term health consequences are beginning to be connected. Overreaching and overtraining are emerging as serious health risks in modern times, in particular with the greatly increased interest in the more extreme endurance sports such as the "Ironman" competitions, tri-athelons and other extreme endurance events. Few athletes who undertake these events are even remotely aware of the massive potential metabolic damage that they may be inflicting on their physiology by failure to consider metabolic stress and taking steps to prevent it.

Fortunately, there is among both the recreational and professional athletic communities a basic understanding of the dangers of overtraining. In the broader non-athletic and largely sedentary community where chronic long term metabolic stress remains largely silent, cardiovascular problems, hypertension and pre-diabetic stress may go unrecognized for years, even decades, apparently tolerated by the unsuspecting masses. However, in both athletic and lay communities, an acute awareness of the potential dangers of suboptimal fueling for exercise and recovery is almost universally lacking. This lack of awareness of the consequences of metabolic damage is most alarming.

Metabolic Stress, Heart Disease in Retired NFL Players

Research by various institutions and investigators in recent years has uncovered other alarming health trends among professional athletes in the U.S. Consider the following facts summarized in a report from the Mayo Clinic in 2008:

- "Retired NFL players are more prone to obesity and obstructive sleep apnea than the general population.

- Retired NFL players have an increased rate of metabolic syndrome, a condition increasingly linked to excess weight and lack of activity, which can lead to Type 2 Diabetes.

- Higher mortality is reported in linemen, as compared to people in the general population of the same age who are not professional football players."[162]

This Mayo Clinic study reported specific concerns linking professional athletes to health risks for cardiovascular disease and stroke. In their study of 233 retired NFL players, aged 35 to 65, researchers found that:

". . .82 percent of NFL players under age 50 had abnormal narrowing and blockages in arteries, compared to the general population of the same age. This finding suggests that the former athletes face increased risk of experiencing high blood pressure, heart attack or stroke. . . The Mayo research team concluded that because test results showed evidence of asymptomatic narrowing of the arteries - called atherosclerosis - the retired NFL players are at abnormally high risk for an adverse cardiovascular event, as compared with people of the same age in the general population. In addition, the high incidence of plaque found in players' vessels suggests that the increased narrowing is not solely due to increased body mass index."[163]

Sounding the Alarm

Preceding the Olympic Games in Atlanta in 1996, a conference was held at the University of Memphis. The purpose was to bring together leading international researchers, physicians and coaches, to discuss the dangers of overtraining in sport. In the book entitled "Overtraining in Sport" published from the conference proceedings, some 84 negative health measures were identified in a chapter by Dr. Mary O'Toole.[164]

Several key measures that can be identified as having strong association with chronic increased metabolic stress include:

Decreased performance, prolonged recovery time, reduced muscle strength, decreased maximum work capacity, changes in blood pressure, elevated metabolic rate, insomnia with and without night sweats, anorexia, loss of appetite, amennhorrhea or oligomenorrhoea, nausea, gastrointestinal disturbances, elevated C-reactive protein, rhabdomyolitis, depression, general apathy, emotional instability, poor concentration during work and training, sensitivity to environmental and emotional stress, decreased capacity to deal with large amounts of information, lack of perserverence ("gives up when the going gets tough"), increased susceptibility to and severity of illness, multiple immune deficits, decreased bone mineral content, mineral depletion, elevated cortisol levels, and low free testosterone.

All of these potentially serious health deficits associated with increased chronic metabolic stress may also be connected to poor liver glycogen status during exercise training and recovery.

It may seem astonishing that in this otherwise excellent book, the liver is virtually ignored. There is no reference to the liver in the extensive index, and no explanation of the critical role of liver glycogen during exercise and recovery. Nor indeed is there any reference to the human brain, its demand for fuel, how this may be compromised during exercise and recovery, and how this may be avoided by optimal fuelling of the liver glycogen store.

Though we concur with the authors regarding the dangers of overtraining in athletics, experience would dictate that most athletes already have a sense of the dangers of this behaviour. What is more obvious is that there is little awareness among trainers and professional athletes of the dangers associated with chronic increased metabolic stress (both hidden and apparent). It is critically essential that all athletes at all levels and of all ages become acutely aware of the deleterious effects of this on exercise training, performance, recovery and long term physiological health.

Athletes of all persuasions must learn how to become HEPATHLETES and consider the benefits of honey, both as a gold standard fuel during exercise (the highest octane fuel on earth), and as a marvelous natural food for selectively refueling the liver during recovery.

8 Honey for Life's Special Conditions and Challenges

Chapter Summary

Honey is therapeutic. The evidence for honey's healthful benefits comes by connecting the dots as follows:

- Honey fuels the liver with adequate glycogen stores
- Liver glycogen fuels the brain
- Inadequate liver glycogen causes the release of glucocorticoids needed to produce alternative fuel for the brain
- Chronic glucocorticoid production is associated with metabolic and intracellular oxidative stress
- Metabolic and intracellular oxidative stress leads to increased risk of many health conditions and diseases
- Eating honey regularly results in reductions in metabolic and intracellular oxidative stress which lowers ones risk for many diseases.

Honey is beneficial for a cascade of conditions & diseases including:

- Diabetes
- Hypertriglyceridemia
- Childhood and adult obesity
- Sleep disorders
- Hypertension
- Gastrointestinal disorders
- Immune system functioning
- Lowering risks for cardiovascular disease and lowering cholesterol
- Hyperhomocysteinemia
- Memory improvement and anxiety reduction
- Improving mental acuity
- Reducing risks for certain forms of cancer
- Dementias, Alzheimer's Disease and other neuro-degenerative conditions
- Liver metabolism and detoxification
- Mental status and depression

Future uses for therapeutic honey may include its use in typhoid fever, resistant tuberculosis and Valley Fever.

Therapeutic Honey

To state that honey can be curative may defy conventional wisdom. But it can be and it is! However, many of the benefits of consuming honey occur over several days, weeks, months or even years in some cases. This may not be good news for a generation hooked on quick fixes, instant cures, immediate gratification and a "can't-I-just-take-a-pill-for-it-Doc?" mentality.

In Chapter 3, we discussed the ways by which honey can be differentiated from sugar or HFCS in terms of observable measurable effects within the body. Over a few weeks or months, honey consumption will prompt lower HbA1c levels in individuals who are pre-diabetic or have full-blown diabetes. In fact, the more advanced one's intolerance for glucose, the better one seems to tolerate honey. This seems counter-intuitive given that honey is equal parts glucose and fructose.

While observational studies have shown us that honey produces a significantly lower elevation in blood sugar levels compared to comparable ingested doses of sucrose or glucose, the physiologic effects of consuming honey versus refined sugar or HFCS may take weeks, months, or even years to be fully revealed. Studies have shown that there is significantly less weight gain in animals fed honey over several months when compared to weight gain in animals fed sucrose or even sugar-free diets.[165] For the same period, triglyceride levels were lower in the honey-fed groups. HDL cholesterol (the good cholesterol) levels were higher indicating that honey also played a role in controlling cholesterol in the honey-fed group.

These results are stunning, however it should be pointed out that the significant differences in blood glucose and HbA1c levels, triglycerides, and HDL cholesterol resulting from the honey diets were not manifested until after several months. In rat years, this translates to mid-life.

In humans, studies that compare dietary variations and their effect on weight typically involve lengthy rigorous protocols with large populations. Randomized controlled studies that compare honey-based diets to diets containing sugar or HFCS would take years to complete. Retrospective studies would be nearly impossible due to the fact that populations not exposed to sugar or HFCS to serve as control groups would be hard to find. However, recent results from short-term human observational studies are very encouraging. Findings indicated that test subjects eating honey *for only 4 weeks*[166] had lower total cholesterol, lower LDL-cholesterol, lower triglycerides, lower fasting blood sugar, and lower C-reactive protein (CRP) while at the same time showing a small reduction in body weight and total body fat.

Connecting the Dots

The good news in all of this is that we do not have to wait for the results of expensive long-term population studies to draw very persuasive conclusions with regard to honey. We know now that the consumption of honey can reduce metabolic stress by refueling the liver. A liver that is kept stocked with glycogen fuels the brain, thus preventing the chronic release of cortisol necessary for the body to convert muscle protein into glucose to fuel the brain. Months and years of metabolic abuse from the release of excessive amounts of cortisol can lead to insulin resistance and hyperglycemia producing intracellular oxidative stress and increased risks for diabetes mellitus, hypertension, cardiovascular disease, osteoporosis, neuro-degenerative diseases such as Alzheimer's Disease and Parkinsonism and contribute to adult and childhood obesity. Honey consumption on a daily, regular basis has a very significant role to play in the prevention of these metabolic diseases and conditions.

Honey can also play a role in reducing intracellular oxidative stress throughout the body. We know that chronically elevated levels of glucose exact a huge toll on the system via damage caused by oxygen free radicals. This damage is most particularly seen in neural or brain tissue. Honey, by virtue of its glucose lowering effects and the small amounts of antioxidants that it contains will combat oxidative stress and prevent and/or reverse over time the effects of free radicals on the aging brain and nervous system.

Honey and Diabetes

There have been countless times in the past couple of years during some occasion in which the authors have been speaking about the health benefits of honey when someone soundly objects, "Oh, I can't eat honey. I have diabetes. My doctor has told me to avoid all sweets." Such, unfortunately, is the state of knowledge about honey among the general public and among most health professionals. Honey and diabetes don't go together.

Rather than arming patients with facts to refute the apparent ignorance of their health care professional – a tactic bound to fail – a better strategy is suggested. Diabetic patients should simply ask their doctor if fruits are permitted in their diets. Since the question is a bit rhetorical, they can have confidence in knowing that honey is permitted. A tablespoon of honey consists of nearly the same carbohydrate content as a cupful of quartered raw apple. The diabetic patient can also be assured that consuming honey will produce a significantly lower blood sugar response than an equivalent amount of sugar or other glucose rich starches.[167]

When consumed regularly over several weeks or months, honey will lower HbA1c levels.[168] Glycosylated (or glycated) hemoglobin, or HbA1c as it is commonly known, is a marker used by physicians to identify the average plasma glucose (blood sugar) concentration over prolonged periods of time. Once glucose becomes attached to the hemoglobin molecule, it remains that way for the life of the red blood cell. The life span of a red blood cell is 120 days. The HbA1c level in the blood can therefore give an indication of the average level of glucose to which the cell has been exposed during its life span. The measurement will be proportional to the average blood glucose concentration during a period of time typically considered to be one to three months prior to the measurement.[169]

From Table 3 that follows, one can see that a small (1%) change in HbA1c levels can represent a significant change in average blood sugar levels.[170] Previously we have observed that honey consumption will result in lower blood sugar levels by as much 60 to 100 mg/dl at 60 and 90 minutes following ingestion of a comparable amount of sucrose.[171] Therefore it is not surprising that the HbA1c levels will be lower by as much as 2 to 4%. *This dietary change alone would mandate tremendous differences in the treatment recommendation guidelines followed by most physicians.* It would no doubt result in much less medicine being prescribed.

Table 3. HbA1c Levels Compared to Average Blood Sugar Levels

HbA1c (%)	Avg. Blood Sugar	
	(mmol/L)	(mg/dL)
4	3.3	60
5	5.0	90
6	6.7	120
7	8.3	150
8	10.0	180
9	11.7	210
10	13.3	240
11	15.0	270
12	16.7	300
13	18.3	330
14	20.0	360

As we have stated before, the more advanced one's glucose intolerance, or in other words the worse their diabetic condition, the greater the positive impact on blood sugar levels from ingesting honey. Logic would dictate that the addition of honey to the diet, along with the elimination of most sugar and

HFCS should be the first recommended treatment of choice for Type 2 Diabetes.

It may surprise most Americans to learn that in many countries around the world that is, in fact, the case.[172, 173] How can this be so and what makes honey so tolerable for those with conditions marked by glucose intolerance? The answer is really quite simple. The balance of sugars and the presence of multiple co-factors in honey serve to make this natural food quite different than table sugar, HFCS or other artificial sweeteners. Honey is an intelligent food, an informed food, a miraculous natural substance!

The physiologic mechanisms responsible for this unique response of the body to honey versus other sugars, HFCS or other starches are not completely understood. The fact that honey does not raise blood sugar levels as does sucrose or HFCS even though it contains the same simple sugars is evidence enough to recommend honey for diabetics.

How much honey is enough? Generally, three to five tablespoons of honey a day is sufficient. A good regimen to follow is to consume a tablespoon or two of honey in the morning with fruit or yogurt or cereal. Another tablespoon should be consumed at bedtime. In between, another one or two tablespoons can be ingested with fruit snacks, in baked goods, or as used in cooking. Honey contains about 60 calories per tablespoon. Generally, the percentage of ones' total caloric requirements provided from simple sugars should not exceed 10%. Thus, the 180 to 300 calories a day provided from honey is sufficient, unless excessive energy demands allow for additional consumption.

Honey and Hypertriglyceridemia

Hypertriglyceridemia is a condition in humans in which triglycerides, the most abundant fatty acid molecule, are chronically elevated above 200 mg/dl. It is found in individuals who chronically consume excessive amounts of sugar, HFCS and even some artificial sweeteners. High triglycerides are also found in those with excessive alcohol intake.

Hypertriglyceridemia is associated with obesity and diabetes mellitus. It is associated with atherosclerosis or plaque development in arteries. Over time, continued high concentrations of triglycerides can lead to pancreatitis.

We have already noted that the consumption of honey, which contains fructose and glucose in nearly equal proportions, does not result in elevations in triglycerides such as are known to occur with the consumption of fructose as found in sucrose or HFCS.[174, 175] This difference though slight and not statistically significant in some studies, further indicates that honey lowers the susceptibility of the heart muscle and coronary blood vessels to peroxidation known to be caused by excess lipids (fats). Honey is actually protective against the oxidative effects of elevated triglycerides.

Honey for Childhood and Adult Obesity

In Chapter 3 we have pointed out the disastrous effects of excessive consumption of refined sugar and HFCS on a generation of children. The association of increased HFCS and sugar consumption with childhood obesity cannot be denied. We have also noted that honey-fed animals gain up to 22% less weight compared to sucrose-fed animals over several months (a period in rats that equates to being middle-aged).[176]

Extrapolation from animal studies to humans is not always exact due to dose and duration of exposure issues. However, one can safely state that a 20+% reduction in weight gain would be a desirable goal for the 20% of the less-than-eighteen-year-old population that are now obese.

There is little doubt that the epidemic of adult obesity has its roots in habits formed at a much younger age. The consumption of honey and the elimination of sugar and HFCS require a definite change of habits. Perhaps more important is the need for education of a generation desperately in need of such a change. Where better to begin an educational program regarding the positive effects of honey than in the early years.

Additionally, we know that honey consumption does not contribute to high blood sugar levels or result in excessive insulin release. In comparison to sugar or HFCS, the differences are significant. The factors that result in an increased risk for insulin resistance, the precursor to diabetes and a host of metabolic diseases, begin at a young age. Common sense would dictate that the consumption of honey during the childhood years along with a sharp reduction in the consumption of HFCS and sucrose would accomplish much in changing the health of a generation.

There is no downside to the substitution of honey for sugar or HFCS! The benefits could be enormous, even revolutionary, if the federally funded school lunch programs in our local public schools adopted such a strategy.

Honey and Hypertension

The association between sleep depravation and elevated blood pressure has been known for some time. Individuals that are deprived of sleep have acutely increased blood pressure which goes along with increased sympathetic nervous system activity. It is thought that repeated and prolonged sleep depravation over several weeks or months could lead to chronic hypertension due to sustained elevations in blood pressure and heart rate and elevated sympathetic nervous system activity.

Recently, Professor James Gangswisch and associates from the School of Public Health at Columbia University in New York, published an article which found that short sleep could be a risk factor for hypertension.[177] In theory then, if one could find an easy drug free way to prolong sleep, one could easily reduce one's risk for hypertension. If one could also reduce the metabolic stress brought on during rest when the brain runs low on fuel, one would reduce catecholamine production that raises blood pressure and heart rate.

Honey does that! In Chapter 5 we have explored in detail the way that honey contributes to and facilitates restorative sleep. Consuming honey before bedtime insures longer sleep by providing needed glycogen to the liver so the brain need not go in search of additional fuel in the early morning hours. Consuming honey before bedtime also reduces the release of adrenalin, a catecholamine that raises blood pressure and heart rate.

Though it cannot be stated categorically that eating honey will reduce one's blood pressure, suggesting honey for hypertension serves as another example of "connecting the dots." Honey promotes restorative sleep, which is defined as improved quality and longer duration sleep. Longer sleep means a reduced risk for hypertension. A reduced risk for hypertension within a population means fewer individuals needing treatment for that widespread condition. The consumption of honey would seem to be a very efficient and cost effective strategy for reducing the risks of hypertension by simply consuming a natural food, a functional food that in the eating, there is no risk.

Honey and Sleep Disorders

Not only does the consumption of honey facilitate and contribute to restorative sleep (Chapter 5), eating honey before bedtime may be a significant aid in combating many of the metabolic abnormalities associated with sleep disorders including sleep apnea. The connection between insufficient sleep and a growing list of metabolic, cardiovascular, and diabetes-related conditions has emerged only in the past five to six years and is something many researchers are vigorously exploring.[178] Yet few in the medical profession or the lay public have yet to connect the dots between insufficient sleep and this cascade of disorders.

Stress due to insufficient sleep (sleep restricted to only 4 hours per night) has been shown to lead to endocrine and metabolic changes associated with insulin resistance, diabetes and weight gain in otherwise healthy young men in as little as one week.[179] Reduced sleep has also been associated with obesity, insulin resistance, and cardiovascular disease in another study.[180] Findings from a large study of over 10,000 civil servants in the United Kingdom indicated that those who reported sleeping only five to seven hours a night had twice the risk of cardiovascular disease.[181]

Metabolic stress is one of the most powerful predictors and risk indicators of disease experienced by contemporary society. Its effects are evidenced in all age groups. We have shown again and again throughout this book that one of the simplest methods of combating metabolic stress is to eat honey regularly. Here again, ***not only does honey have a role to play in reducing*** *metabolic stress, but it also will help prevent occurrences of insufficient sleep, an emerging cause of many metabolic conditions.*

Honey and Gastrointestinal Disorders

In Chapter 9, the antimicrobial effects of honey will be discussed in more detail. Here, we simply call attention to the potential role that consuming honey can play in combating many gastrointestinal disorders. Many cases of peptic ulcers, gastritis, duodenitis, and cancers are caused by the bacteria *Helicobacter pylori* (*H. pylori*). Antibiotics prescribed for *H. pylori* infections are expensive and frequently produce side effects while destroying normal gastrointestinal bacteria. Honey is a very effective antibacterial agent (killing even resistant strains of some bacteria) at concentrations as low as five to fifteen percent. Perhaps the best news is that honey has no side effects. It can be eaten regularly without risk.

Honey is also a very effective probiotic, meaning that it contains potentially beneficial bacteria such as Lactobacillus and Bifidobacterium[182] and other residual compounds associated with these bacteria. Several research studies have confirmed the positive effects of probiotics on gastrointestional health. These are summarized in the text box below.

Beneficial Effects of Probiotics

* Improvement and management of lactose Intolerance
* Prevention of colon cancer
* Lowered cholesterol
* Lowered blood pressure
* Improvment in immune system functioning
* Prevention of infections from H. pylori
* Relieve antibiotic-associated diarrhea
* Reduce Inflammation
* Improved mineral absorption from the gastrointestinal tract
* Prevention of harmful bacterial growth under stress
* Relieve irritable bowel syndrome (IBS) and colitis symptoms

Honey for Oral Health, Gingivitis, Periodontal Disease, and Radiation-induced Mucositis

Many conditions affecting oral health, including dental caries, gingivitis and periodontal disease are caused by bacteria which normally reside in the mouth. Honey can be an effective agent in controlling these bacteria because of its potent antibiotic actions.

The use of honey for this purpose comes with a possible downside, however. Honey is very acidic and if left in contact with tooth enamel for any prolonged period of time will erode the enamel. Therefore, when consuming undiluted honey it is a good idea to rinse the mouth with water afterwords to prevent damage to tooth enamel.

In two separate studies in Egypt and Iran, honey has also been found to be helpful in both preventing and managing the damage caused to mucosal membranes in the mouth secondary to radiation treatments.[183, 184] Patients with head and neck cancers receiving radiation treatments frequently have what is known as radiation-induced mucositis. Honey treatments provided simple economic relief without side effects.

Honey and Enhanced Immune System Functioning

Clinical and laboratory studies have demonstrated that regular consumption of honey results in elevation of platelet counts, stabilization of hemoglobin levels, and improvements in white blood cell counts, all results that are associated with improved immune system functioning.[185, 186] One of the more amazing evidences of honey's potential role in immune system enhancement comes from a study involving the use of a special type of honey (known as LifeMel Honey or LMH) in the treatment of cancer patients.

These results were described in a paper by Dr. Jamal Zidon and his associates who reported on a study conducted at several hospitals in Israel on severely ill cancer patients with multiple types of cancers. These patients all had acute febrile neutropenia (AFN), a life-threatening condition in which the white blood cell counts are dangerously low. All of the patients required treatment with Colony Stimulating Factor (CSF), an expensive drug given to boost the immune system response.

The patients, all being treated with various chemotherapy protocols, were given, in addition, a teaspoon of LMH honey for five days before their second round of chemotherapy doses. Remarkably, there was no recurrence of neutropenia after the honey treatment. 40% of the patients had no need for additional CSF treatments. Most patients included in the study group showed increased neutrophil counts, decreased occurrences of thrombocytopenia (low platelet count), and stabilized hemoglobin levels at >11 grams/dl.

These findings are consistent with other published reports citing the immune system enhancement effects of honey however no specific biochemical mechanisms were given to explain the results.

Honey for Lowering Cholesterol and Reducing Other Risk Factors for Cardiovascular Disease

A recent study published in early 2008 found that ingestion of 70 grams of natural honey a day for only 30 days reduced several risk factors for cardiovascular disease in overweight or obese human subjects when compared to ingestion of 70 grams of sucrose.[187] Subjects eating honey had lower total cholesterol, lower LDL-cholesterol, lower triglycerides, lower fasting blood sugar, and lower C-reactive protein (CRP) while at the same time showing a small reduction in body weight and total body fat. These findings, though from a small human study group (55 patients) and not all statistically significant, are still remarkable and provide confirmation of the potential role for honey in combating the risk of cardiovascular disease in populations already at risk.

Another small limited human observational study completed in 2003 demonstrated that natural unprocessed honey consumed daily for 15 days lowered thromboxane (B2) and two different prostaglandin (PGE2 and PGF2a) levels in normal individuals by 48, 63 and 50% respectively.[188]

Prostaglandins, in the human system, together with the thromboxanes form a class of fatty acid derivatives which are potent "mediators" of a variety of strong physiological effects. They are technically hormones, although they are rarely classified as such. In general, prostaglandins are thought of as mediators of inflammation in the body. Both prostaglandins and thromboxanes have been implicated in immune system suppression and atherosclerosis, an underlying cause of cardiovascular disease. To the degree that honey lowers prostaglandin levels when consumed regularly over time, it would appear from this study that honey can reduce the risks of cardiovascular disease.

Honey and Hyperhomocysteinemia

Most of us have never heard of hyperhomocysteinemia. We do however know something about the effect of elevated levels of this amino acid in humans. In some individuals, elevated levels of homocysteine accumulate and pose an imminent threat to ones heart and blood vessels. Homocysteine (HCY) is a normal by-product of metabolism of the amino acid, methionine. When HCY accumulates, the condition is known as hyperhomocysteinemia and is associated with an increased risk of heart disease, osteoporosis and Alzheimer's disease, presumably due to the effects of oxidative damage. About 10% of the coronary related deaths each year are attributed to abnormally high levels of HCY.

In a study published in 2006, it was demonstrated that consumption of natural honey had a significant lowering effect on homocysteine.[189] The study results indicated that honey in only a 1% solution fed to rats improved growth, and provided protection against elevated homocysteine levels. This is another stunning example of honey metabolism and its physiologic effects not available from the consumption of other refined sugars such as sucrose and high fructose corn syrup.

Honey and Memory Improvement and Anxiety Reduction

One of the more exciting benefits of honey relates to its potential role in memory performance or enhancement. Many investigations over the past fifteen years or so have demonstrated the effects of hormones, specifically cortisol, on the hippocampus, a part of the brain belonging to the limbic system and responsible for memory and spatial navigation.[190, 191, 192, 193] Both animal and human studies have shown that metabolic stress from excessive cortisol levels is responsible for memory impairment, by causing both neuronal excitability and eventual cell loss. These results are consistent across a variety of conditions that result in excessive glucocorticoid (cortisol) levels. Spatial memory deficits, deficits in verbal recall, and increases in anxiety have been observed in patients with Cushing's syndrome who are taking therapeutic doses of steroids.[194, 195] In a lengthy review that focused on the hormonal changes associated with pregnancy, the patterns of memory loss both during and after pregnancy indicated the cause as being hippocampal dysfunction. Pregnancy is known to be associated with elevated levels of cortisol.[196] These same deficits have also been observed in animals given excessive doses of synthetic glucocorticoids. In both volunteers and patients with Cushing's syndrome, memory performance improved with reduction in the excess glucocorticoid.[197, 198]

Regular daily consumption of honey has a direct effect on the levels of cortisol produced in the body. Honey is the ideal food for fueling the liver which is the primary fuel store for the brain. When the liver glycogen stores remain adequate for brain function, circulating cortisol levels remain lower. Cortisol is not released in an attempt to provide backup fuel for the brain. It really is that simple! Regular honey consumption prevents the chronic and excessive release of cortisol which is the principle cause of metabolic stress. Chronic metabolic stress caused by increased cortisol levels impacts memory by damaging hippocampal neurons.

In one rather elegant animal study referenced earlier,[199] rats fed honey over a twelve month period were observed to have better spacial memory and reduced anxiety as compared to those fed a sucrose diet. The authors speculated that as different areas of the hippocampus mediate these behaviors and these areas are susceptible to oxidative damage over time, honey may have been responsible for the positive results because of its antioxidant content. As stated, honey has an effect on preventing excess cortisol release. It seems perfectly reasonable to state therefore, that the consumption of honey can prevent memory degradation and lessen anxiety by its role in limiting cortisol production and release (the primary cause of metabolic stress) and by providing antioxidants necessary to reverse oxidative damage.

Honey and Mental Acuity

It is one thing to observe improvements or changes in memory function in laboratory animals given dietary changes (honey versus sucrose) over time as in the study referenced in the above section. It is quite another to experience the transient dip in mental acuity common to many of us in the early to mid-afternoon consistant with a falling blood glucose as a result of insulin release in the post-lunch period. It is yet another to find that cognitive impairment or decline in cognitive ability such as seen in dementias, Alzheimer's disease, and other neuro-degenerative conditions is frequently associated with diabetes or chronic impairments in blood glucose.

What about the observations that link poor classroom performance and lack of attentiveness with missing a good morning breakfast? Or the repeated cycles of a quick sugar "fix" followed by a lethargic phase experienced in young people who consume canned sodas throughout the day. Or the professional soccer players (footballers in the UK and Europe) who fuel up on sugar cakes and high calorie sugary drinks at half time and experience sluggish performance, slowed raction times, increased penalties, and poor concentration during the second half.

David Beckham, now a familiar American sports icon, experienced just such a "second half hypoglycemia" in a 2006 World Cup soccer match when England played Ecuador. The English soccer coaches are still at a loss to explain why their last two World Cup teams performed so badly, expecially in the second half of critical matches. Had they eaten honey at half time and thereby refueled the liver and provided for a stable blood glucose during the second half, it is fair to say they may have maintained a sharpened mental acuity and performed to potential.

The universal "liver blindness" in sports contributed to their poor results in spite of their high levels of skill and the optimism of their fans. In addition, chronic over-secretion of insulin from high sugar content snacks stimulates sympathoadrenal hormone activity causing increased blood pressure and increased heart rate, none of which can be considered conducive to optimal brain functioning or consistant athletic performance.

In cases where the drinks contain artificial sweeteners, the resulting experience may be even more acute. Insulin release via the gustatory effect that occurs with the consumption of these drinks will drive down blood glucose levels without an initial rise in blood glucose and the outcome will again be poor mental acuity.

Is there a metabolic phenomenon or causative thread that ties all of these observations together? We think there is. Scientific research is beginning to connect the dots.

Diabetes provides us with a window through which impaired mental acuity has been observed and linked in some cases to episodes of hypoglycemia. In other cases, observations have suggested that cognitive impairment or reduction in cognitive ability may occur with or withour hypoglycemia. One study of patients with insulin dependent diabetes mellitus (IDDM) linked poor cognitive ability with chronic hypoglycemia, showing a "significant association between a history of recurrent severe hypoglycemia and cortical atrophy which may be related to the modest impairment of cognitive function that has been reported previoulsly."[200] However the results from another study just two years later in 1999, reported seemingly contradictory results indicating that "repeated episodes of hypoglycaemia were not related to cognitive decrement, and initial mental ability was not associated with eventual numbers of hypoglycaemic episodes in this group of patients."[201]

The question arises - how can we explain cognitive impairment in diabetic patients where this decline in cognitive ability is not directly linked to episodes of hypoglycaemia? This may be explained if we look a little more in depth into neural cell metabolism as well as metabolic stress throughout the system.

Mental Acuity in Hypo- and Hyperglycemia

During an acute episode of hypoglycaemia, blood glucose falls rapidly and glucose supply to the brain is compromised. This is a well documented aspect of such an episode, and most of us have experienced this at some time in our lives. Thoughts become confused and muddled and reaction times slowed. Another example of an acute stress response occurs in marathon runners near the end of a race in which they may often become so confused that they scarcely know where they are, or indeed who they are. During this acute stress response, blood pressure rises, heart rate increases, temperature rises causing sweats and in some cases shakes and even colapse.

Chronic stress may manifest itself differently. Chronic or repeatedly elevated cortisol levels in neurons or brain cells will inhibit glucose metabolism and disposal, just the same as what takes place in muscle cells. Intracellular glucose concentrations will rise creating a situation where fuel supply in neurons is high but utilization of that fuel is impaired. Neuronal cell functions including cognitive ability and thought processes are compromised.

In other words a drop in glucose supply as in acute episodes of hypoglycemia may have the same metabolic outcome as chronically increased glucose concentrations that occur over time due to impaired glucose metabolism. Both hypoglycemia and hyperglycemia result in functional deficits in critical fuel supply to brain cells resulting in cognitive deficits.

This latter chronic form of impairment in mental acuity resulting from increased glucose concentration within neural cells may be termed a form of "cerebral diabetes." The various neuronal metabolic conditions expressed are the result of compromised glucose metabolism and linked to break down of energy pathways and energy management in brain cells in different regions of the brain. The long term result of such chronically raised metabolic stress in brain cells is all too clear and tragic - memory loss, dementias, Alzheimer's disease and other neuro-degenerative conditions.

It seems surprising that a simple natural food such as honey eaten at critical times will provide protection against these conditions. By optmally fuelling the liver, we fuel the brain and reduce metabolic stress in neural tissues and thereby optimise cognitive function. To ignor this simple solution seems foolish indeed.

Honey and Depression

The causes of clinical depression are varied and include factors from three broad categories: psychological, physiological and environmental. The focus in this book has been on the physiologic or metabolic stress as opposed to the psychological or environmental. However, stress from whatever the cause is universally associated with elevations in glucocorticoid release. The link between elevated cortisol levels and anxiety and depression has been established in several studies.[202, 203, 204]

In a wonderful book called *The Human Motor*, Anson Rabinach describes a classic experiment carried out in the early 20th century, on mental fatigue in students.[205] A German researcher, Wilhelm Weichardt, entered a classroom, armed with sprayers containing a 1% solution called "antikenotoxin" (anti-fatigue vaccine) and sprayed the vaccine into the atmosphere. The students were informed that the spray would improve the air quality. In the afternoon the students were given tests and although already fatigued, the results were extraordinary. Calculation speeds improved by 50% and errors were reduced. Some of the students seemed fresher than they had been in the morning.

One may ask just what does this have to do with depression. Depression, as we have stated, may be from psychological, metabolic or environmental causes. Mental fatigue and psycological stress within the classroom contribute to elevations in cortisol levels which in turn inhibit glucose metabolism in cells, specifically brain cells. Here we have an explanation for Weichardt's anti-fatigue spray. The suggestion of improved air qualtiy apparently had a positive impact on the student's psychological state which would have modulated stress physiology, and thus improved brain function and test performance. Reduced production and release of adrenal stress hormones results in lower levels of cortisol in neurones. The outcome in neural processing may have resulted in improved memory recall and mental acuity.

This anecdotal evidence gives us another example of the interrelationship between stress physiology, memory, and mental acuity described by Dinan in 1994.[206] We have also seen how low levels of liver glycogen result in increased physiologic stress and negatively impact mental acuity. It follows that selective restocking of the liver glycogen stores at critical times with honey will minimize this metabolic stress.

Depression provides us with another example of the interrelationship between physiological and psychological stress. Depression is known to be associated with defects in the central nervous system's cortisol receptors. This "downgrading" results in reactivation of the negative feedback signals required to reduce glucocorticoid levels. Pharmacological agents used in the treatment of depression known as tricyclic anti-depressants and selective serotonin re-uptake inhibitors (SSRIs) reverse this stress induced deficiency of serotonin in the presynaptic space, in effect increasing the level of neurotransmitters present. Lopez in a paper published in 1998 confirmed these findings and demonstrated again the connection between depression and chronic hypercortisolism or cortisol driven metabolic stress.[207]

Another excellent example of the modulatory dynamics that occur in depression comes from patients who suffer from Cushing's syndrome, a disease that results from chronic overproduction of cortisol or hypercortisolism. These individuals are at high risk of depression.[208] However, when the cortisol levels are returned to normal, the depression is relieved.

In Chapter 5, we described the SCN in the hippocampal region of the brain and its role in metabolism and sleep regulation. The hippocampus is the region of the brain most at risk from cortisol excess. The hippocampus serves as the short term memory bank. Here again we have powerful links between metabolic stress from elevated cortisol levels, memory processing and depression.[209]

Also in Chapter 5, we indicated how the activity of 11BetaHSD-1, an enzyme rich in the brain, is responsible for converting inactive cortisone into active intracellular cortisol.[210] We noted that by simply maintaining liver glycogen stores, one could limit the activation of this enzyme and thus reduce the effects of cortisol activation. Here again, we can link improved liver glycogen status by ingestion of honey to improved neural processing and in turn to a positive impact on depression by decreasing cortisol levels.

It is interesting to note that much research is being done currently with regard to cortisol antagonists as potential treatment for severe depression. How much easier to simply take a little honey!

Honey and Dementias, Alzheimer's Disease and Other Neuro-degenerative Conditions

Previously we have discussed how hyperglycemia or chronic high blood sugar levels eventually causes irreversible damage to the brain through an increase in free radical generation (Chapter 3, pages 30, 31). One way of describing this situation is as a form of *cerebral diabetes* in which glucose metabolism is compromised and proteins are attacked to provide alternative fuel. Chronic metabolic stress is the key causative event. The combination of impaired glucose metabolism and decreasing antioxidant production in the body as we age, results in brain cell damage.

Honey consumption as we have shown will lower glucose levels thus reducing the risk of impaired glucose metabolism over time. In addition, honey provides small amounts of antioxidants necessary to reverse the destructive effects of free radicals on the aging brain and nervous system. *Prevention* of oxidative damage associated with the several complications of diabetes and the progression of other age related conditions such as Alzheimer's disease, vascular dementias, Parkinsonism, memory and cognition loss is much simpler than treatment. Lifelong excessive consumption of sugar and HFCS is known to be associated with all of these conditions. The regular consumption of honey, by virtue of its ability to regulate blood sugar by lowering circulating blood sugar levels and to reduce oxidative stress, seems to be a sweet simple solution that will mitigate the risks of these diseases and prevent their occurrences.

Honey and Liver Metabolism and Detoxification

One of the best kept secrets of honey metabolism is the ability of this amazing food to facilitate in the detoxification of alcohol and protect the liver from toxic damage associated with alcohol consumption. While we are not in any way attempting to justify or excuse excess alcohol consumption, it would be advised to consider the facts presented in this section the next time you have a few drinks.

Repeatedly throughout this book we have focused on the role of honey as an ideal source of liver glycogen which is available to fuel the brain during times when the brain is at greatest risk from low fuel reserves such as during exercise and sleep. Another time when the brain is at risk is during and immediately following the consumption of alcohol.

Alcohol is a powerful oxidant. It is detoxified primarily in the liver. When consumed it forces the liver into immediate action to combat potential damage from free radical accumulation. In addition, alcohol has a hypoglycemic effect on the system, driving down blood glucose levels. When drinking excessively, brain metabolism slows, cognitive function declines, speech becomes slurred and incoherent and the resultant extreme metabolic stress of continued alcohol intake may lead to coma, expecially in young people.

The enzyme responsible for detoxifying alcohol in the liver is alcohol dehydrogenase. Alcohol is first converted to acetaldehyde and then to acetic acid by the action of this enzyme. Both reactions use up stores of the enzyme nicotinomide adenine dinucleotide (NAD) which is reduced to NADH. NAD is the rate limiting factor in the pathway of alcohol detoxification.

As we have stated in Chapter 3, fructose from excess refined sugar and HFCS consumption is associated with many adverse health consequences.

However fructose, if consumed in reasonable quantity is central to human energy metabolsm. Fructose as supplied in honey is critical in maintaining fuel supply for the hungry brain during those periods when brain metabolism is most at risk - exercise and during the night fast. Fructose also comes to the rescue of a stressed liver and recycles the reduced enzyme NADH back to NAD, restarting the cycle and allowing for more alcohol to be detoxified.[211] In addition, honey is packed with a wonderful array of antioxidants which will provide protection against the free radical attack on liver and other cells in the body.

Several papers published by Dr. Noori Al-Waili have demonstrated the protective benefits of honey consumption on the liver. In one, levels of glutathione reductase were shown to be increased. Glutathione reductase is a powerful antioxidant form of glutathione and is one of the most important antioxidant enzymes in the body and vital to liver function.[212] In another, honey provided protection against liver cell damage from exposure to a substance known to be toxic to the liver cells. The author concluded that "exclusive honey feeding (50% concentration) significantly modifies and ameliorates biochemical and hematological changes . . ."[213]

The next time you are thinking about potentially harming your liver with alcohol consumption, be wise and take a tablespoon of natural honey before and after you drink. You will do your liver and yourself a favor.

Honey and Reduced Cancer Risks

Honey is a potent stimulant of the immune system in humans by virtue of both direct and indirect mechanisms. The consumption of honey directly stimulates the production of immune factors within the system. Honey also acts indirectly by inhibiting metabolic stress, reducing the production of cortisol in particular. Cortisol is one of the most powerful hormone inhibitors of immune function.

In the study by Dr. Zidon referenced on page 127 above, a significant reversal of immune system collapse in patients receiving chemotherapy was observed following the ingestion of a specialized form of honey. Improving immunity in cancer not only reduces risk of opportunist infections, but provides immune ammunition against cancer cells. Other animal studies have provided tantalizing suggestions of a more direct influence on carcinogenesis, resulting from honey consumption.[214]

It is not to be inferred from this that any person with cancer may be cured by consuming honey. However, we are suggesting that honey when consumed as a natural sweetener may play a role in cancer prevention, something that cannot be said about all other refined sugars and artificial sweeteners. One of the more intriguing aspects of natural plant bioflavonoids, something not found in sugar or HFCS, is that when they exhibit anti-diabetic activity, they also are found to have significant anti-carcinogenic activity.[215]

This should not be as surprising as it seems at first glance. Observations of cancer cells and diabetic cells indicate that they share one major similarity, that of impaired mitochondrial activity.[216] Within a normal cell, a 6-carbon glucose molecule is metabolized anaerobically (without oxygen) to 3-carbon pyruvate. The 3-carbon pyruvate is then transferred into the mitochondria where it is oxidized to carbon dioxide and water with the release of energy. In the diabetic cell, glucose is not stored as glycogen and may not be transferred into the mitochondria for oxidation. In other words, glucose is not disposed of normally. As the intracellular concentration of glucose rises, preventing new glucose from entering the cell, blood glucose concentration rises.

In the cancer cell the mitochondria also malfunction. However, the clever cancer cell hyper-activates or accelerates the first stage of glucose metabolism into pyruvate. Pyruvate is then converted to lactic acid which is then metabolized as fuel. This process is less efficient than normal glucose metabolism and uses up huge quantities of glucose with less energy production. The result is that lean body tissue (protein) must now be degraded to create new glucose and feed the cancer.

Some recent cancer therapies have focused on mechanisms that reactivate the malfunctioning mitochondria. Some plant bioflavonoids appear to have the ability to do this. Once the mitochondria is able to function normally, it may then activate apoptosis (cell suicide) and the cancer cell dies. This is the most likely mechanism whereby these active plant principles express anti-carcinogenic activity. Research studies are ongoing in many laboratories around the world.

Researchers at the University of Dundee, Scotland have uncovered the putative pathway by which these bioflavonoids may act. Their work first suggested that metformin (Glucophage), the most popular anti-diabetic drug prescribed in the United States, exhibited a potential anti-carcinogenic effect. [217] Metformin, a drug from the biguanide class of drugs originating from the French lilac plant, is used to improve insulin signaling in diabetes and had been known to reduce cancer risk in diabetic patients taking this drug. The drug is now emerging as a potential treatment for patients with some forms of cancer.[218]

Metformin works by increasing insulin sensitivity, enhancing peripheral glucose uptake and inhibiting gluconeogenesis (the formation of glucose from amino acids) in the liver, thereby lowering blood glucose levels overall. That it reduces cancer risk should not be surprising. We know that there are over 100,000 obesity related cancer deaths each year in the United States. Metformin is very effective in the treatment of Type 2 Diabetes, especially in individuals with accompanying obesity and insulin resistance.

When insulin signaling is improved, glucose metabolism and disposal within the cell is improved and normal mitochondrial functioning is restored.

Cancer risks are reduced. The incidence of some forms of cancer is reduced simply by correcting glucose metabolism and disposal. This link, now being confirmed in additional research, underscores the need to control and/or limit metabolic stress not only to reduce the morbidity from Type 2 Diabetes and obesity but for some forms of cancer as well.

When considering the many bio-active principles in honey that improve glucose metabolism and disposal via improved insulin signaling, plus the trace amounts of vitamins, minerals, amino acids, bioflavonoids, organic acids, nitric oxide, hydrogen peroxide and other volatiles, one begins to appreciate the reasons why the consumption of honey, as compared to other refined sugars, may reduce risk of some forms of cancer. HFCS and artificial sweeteners have none of the insulin signaling principles of honey. Consumption of these sugars and sweeteners result in the release of excessive amounts of insulin and eventually hyperinsulinism, insulin resistance and increased risk of cancers due to impaired mitrochondrial function. Honey reduces the amount of insulin release due to its balanced fructose/glucose content and its improved insulin signaling. Honey acts as "proto-insulin" which in effect reduces the requirement for insulin and improves glucose metabolism and disposal.

This fact alone may prove to be one of the great unsung, key secrets of natural honey, a wonderful energy boosting food that improves insulin signaling activity without the benefit of insulin. On the surface this appears to be a contradiction. Closer scrutiny indicates that this observation has potent implications for human nutrition. The powerful health message is that consumption of honey may reduce the risks of cancer by reducing metabolic stress and improving glucose metabolism. The evidence is growing. The simple message is clear and compelling.

By joining the Honey Revolution, and reducing the consumption of refined sugars and HFCS in favor of honey, overall health can be improved, and the risks of metabolic diseases, including some forms of cancers can be reduced. Certainly there is no risk in trying.

Honey and Allergies

Perhaps the most frequently asked question pertaining to the healthful benefits of consuming honey is "Will eating local honey help my allergies?" For decades, it has been a belief of many that exposure to small doses of pollen contained in honey will help desensitize one to particular allergens and reduce allergic symptoms. Where better to find small doses of pollens than in honey produced from the local region where one lives.

There are a couple of challenges to this belief that need to be mentioned. First of all, this is probably one of the most researched aspects of potential health benefits from honey reported in the scientific literature. The results have been rather non-conclusive for a number of reasons, including the number of confounding variables associated with the allergic phenomenon, the lack of adequate control groups, and the complexity of the body's immune responses. The FDA does not allow pollen marketers in the United States to make health claims about their product as no scientific basis for these claims has ever been proved. However much anecdotal evidence continues to support the theory that eating "local" honey will help reduce one's allergic responses.

The second issue relates to the nature of allergens produced by plant and tree pollen. Most pollen found in honey is of the type known as entomophilous, that is pollen dispersed by animals or insects. This pollen is heavier and stickier and does not typically become airborne. Most flower producing plants frequented by honeybees produce this type of pollen which is usually not associated with allergic reactions in humans. Generally pollens that cause allergies in humans are those of anemophilous plants which produce a light, dry pollen that is dispersed by air currents over a wide region. Such plants produce large quantities of this lightweight pollen which when airborne and can be easily inhaled and come into contact with the sensitive mucous membranes in the nose resulting in typical allergic reactions.

There is no scientific proof that honey will help your allergies, however there is certainly no evidence that it will make them worse. This is one of those areas in which eating honey will do no harm, but is cannot be stated unequivocally that it will help.

Future Uses of Therapeutic Honey

Currently there are several studies being conducted in various parts of the world in university and other research centers which are seeking to discover the exact properties of honey responsible for other health or medicinal benefits. The next couple of years hold promise of more discoveries. It would not be surprising to see many more ways in which honey will be found healthful and therapeutic. Following are a few examples.

Honey for Typhoid Fever

Pakistini researchers have demonstrated that black seed honey produced in that country has the ability in low concentrations (7%-16%) to inhibit growth of typhoidal salmonellae isolated from typhoid patients.[219] Simulated honey used as a control at concentrations up to 25% did not inhibit any typhoid isolate in vitro. This study indicates just one of the potential applications available for honey and recommends its continued evaluation in animal and human research.

Honey for Tuberculosis and Valley Fever

To date, the authors know of patent applications in at least three countries for the use of honey delivered via nebulizer for use in respiratory diseases, tuberculosis, and coccidioidomycosis (also known as Valley Fever, San Joaquin Valley Fever, California Valley Fever, or desert fever). There are several reasons why this use of honey may prove to be significant in these conditions. Inhalation from a nebulizer directly into the lungs is a very effective way of delivering medication. The mucosal lining of the lungs is a very vascular-rich membrane which rapidly absorbs inhaled medications. Nebulized delivery of honey would place the effective antimicrobial agent directly in contact with the infective organizm. The delivery of honey via a nebulizer has been tested in human subjects. Results have shown that honey concentrations up to 60% do not cause adverse reactions nor do they have any significant impact on blood sugar levels.[220]

In vitro laboratory studies have found that honey is a very effective antibiotic against the tuberculosis mycobacteria, including the highly resistant strains, even at concentrations less than 20%.[221, 222] The continued spread of drug-resistant strains of TB from Mexico into the U.S. is creating concern for U.S. health officials.[223] It follows that nebulized honey delivered in concentrations of between 10% and 20% would be effective against these orgainsms.

To the authors knowledge, honey has not been tested against coccidioidomycosis, however honey has been found to be effective against other fungal organisms in concentrations of less than 30%. The expense of this type of treatment would be a fraction of the typical cost of the pharmaceuticals now used to combat these infections. Clinical and laboratory tests must, of course, be conducted to insure the efficacy of honey in these diseases, but it is difficult to find a disadvantage or downside to this therapeutic use of honey.

9 Honey That Soothes and Heals

Summary

The use of honey as an antimicrobial dates to antiquity. For centuries, honey has been used as an effective treatment against many types of bacteria, including resistant organisms and some fungi.

The active ingredient in honey responsible for its potent antibiotic activity has been identified as methylglyoxal. Honey that contains methylglyoxal should be consumed with caution, especially for those who have diabetes or impaired glucose tolerance.

Honey is also an effective cough suppressant in children. Comparative studies have found it to be more effective than dextromethorphan, the leading OTC drug used in most cough syrups.

Honey as an Effective Anti-microbial

The use of honey as a topical treatment for wounds, burns, and infections has been documented in recorded history dating back to before 2000 BC in Egyptian writings. The text box which follows includes just a few of the many references from antiquity regarding the medicinal use of honey.

Two and a half centuries ago, Dr. John Hill, a physician from England wrote:

> "The slight regard at this time paid to the medicinal virtues of Honey, is an instance of neglect men shew to common objects, whatever their value: acting in contempt, as it were, of the immediate hand of providence, which has in general made those things most frequent, which have the greatest uses; and for that reason, we seek from the remotest part of the world, medicines of harsh and violent operation for our relief in several disorders, under which we should never suffer, if we would use what the Bee collects for us at our doors."[224]

John Hill, MD (1759)

Medicinal Uses of Honey in the Recorded History of Many Cultures

2100 - 2000 B.C. - The Sumerians mixed river dust with honey and oil to treat infected skin ulcers - a prescription written on clay tablets.

About 2000 B.C. - The Egyptians used honey to treat open wounds.

1800 B.C. - The Babylonians used honey in medicine and referred to it in the Code of Hammurabi.

1400 B.C. - Sustra, a surgeon from India wrote of the medicinal properties of eight different honey varietals.

1200 B.C. - Charak, another Indian physician regarded honey as a tonic and a mild laxative.

230 A.D. - Athenaeus from Ancient Greece wrote that all who ate honey and bread for breakfast "were free from disease all their lives."

About 650 A.D. - Ibn Magih, from the Arab-Muslim culture quoted from Mohammed in writing "honey is a remedy for every illness."

600 - 700 AD - The Chinese mixed honey with opium as a therapeutic relief for pain.

1759 - the first English book on honey was published by Sir John Hill. "The Virtues of Honey in Preventing many of the worst Disorders, and in the Certain Cure of Several others . . ."

[All references taken from *Honey A Comprehensive Survey,* edited by Eva Crane, MSc, PhD, Crane, Russak & Company, Inc., New York, Printed in Great Britain, 1975]

Twenty-first century science has confirmed what the ancients believed and what men throughout the centuries have known experientially and intuitively. Honey is therapeutic. When applied as a topical antibiotic, honey's healing properties cover a wide range of infective agents. Researchers from New Zealand and Australia have lead the way in the study of honey and its antibiotic potential for decades. Perhaps best of all, the use of honey in this manner comes without side effects.

In 2002, Joe Traynor published a wonderful treatise entitled "Honey The Gourmet Medicine."[225] In his book, Traynor documents that the effectiveness of honey in destroying bacteria comes from at least four properties found in various honey varietals. All four properties are not found in all honey varietals to the same degree.

Four Anti-microbial Properties of Honey

First of all honey is hyperosmolar - that is, its water content is very low, generally below eighteen percent. When in contact with other tissues, honey literally absorbs water from cells, killing them.

Second, honey is very acidic. The pH of honey averaged across many varietals is less than 4.0 making it more acidic than most foods and even some acids. Low acidity inhibits the growth of most bacteria.

Third, honey has the ability to generate hydrogen peroxide under certain conditions. Hydrogen peroxide has been used as a disinfectant for decades, but because it is unstable in the presence of light and air, it is difficult to store and utilize. Hydrogen peroxide in high concentrations is also quite toxic to human tissue making it less attractive as a topical disinfectant. Honey solves this dilemma and provides an ideal mechanism for producing hydrogen peroxide in controlled amounts.

Honey contains the enzyme glucose oxidase. This enzyme comes from the honeybee's stomach and small amounts of it remain in honey as it is extracted, processed and packed for resale. Glucose oxidase works on the glucose in honey, breaking it down into gluconic acid and hydrogen peroxide. However, the enzyme is not active in pure honey because of its low pH and low sodium content. Activation of glucose oxidase requires a pH of at least 5.5 and a sodium content of at least 2300 parts per million (ppm). The sodium content of pure honey is only 20 to 40 ppm.

Honey when applied to a burn, wound or infected tissue begins to work its wonders only as serum from the tissues dilutes the honey raising its pH and adding sodium thus activating glucose oxidase. The action of glucose oxidase delivers small controlled portions of hydrogen peroxide directly to the site of an infection or wherever honey is applied. Thus, the miracle of pure honey is its hydrogen peroxide generating *potential*. Traynor summarizes this capability of honey with these words:

"Thus, minute doses of hydrogen peroxide are continually released from the honey, directly to where they are most needed. Could man devise a more perfect, slow-release antimicrobial product for treating wounds? If a billion dollar, biomedical company gave their research and development scientists unlimited time and resources, it is doubtful they could equal what nature has already provided in honey. It's enough to make even the most skeptical scientist believe in a higher being, as if God, in His wisdom, provided man with a perfect elixir to treat wounds and infections. Doctors in the U.S., with rare exceptions, have rejected this gift."[226]

This potential ability to produce hydrogen peroxide is not found in all honey, however. Some honey even contains small quantities of the enzyme catalase. Catalase neutralizes hydrogen peroxide, thus diminishing the effectiveness of honey as an antimicrobial.

Fourth, honey contains other floral factors obtained from nectar. One of these is a recently discovered ingredient in honey known as methylglyoxal (MGO). MGO is perhaps related to what Peter Molan from New Zealand has called the Unique Manuka Factor or UMF found in higher concentrations in Manuka honey made from the flowers of the Manuka bush in New Zealand.

In January of 2008, Professor Thomas Henle, head of the Institute of Food Chemistry at the Technical University of Dresden, published an article in which he refers to the results of a Dresden study which "unambiguously demonstrates for the first time that methylglyoxal is directly responsible for the antibacterial activity of Manuka Honey."[227] Researchers at the university analyzed 40 samples of honey from various sources around the world, including New Zealand honeys. They found methylglyoxal levels in Manuka honeys were up to 1000-fold higher than non-manuka products.

The important fact to note in this discussion is that all honey, regardless of the varietal, possesses some of the properties that make honey effective against bacteria. Multiple varietals of honey were tested by Dr. Shona Blair and her associates from the University of Sydney in Australia. Though there was wide variation among varietals as to their effectiveness as an antimicrobial among the honey used in their study, effective mean concentrations (Mean Inhibitory Concentration or MIC) of honey varied from just 2-16% when applied against the more than 60 problematic pathogens studied.[228] These pathogens included several antibiotic resistant micro-organisms, many species of anaerobic bacteria, Candida and Tinea fungi, and biofilms (microorganisms that secrete a slimy protective coating that makes them resistant to antibiotics). Sugar solutions used as controls in this study required mean concentrations of >20 to 45% to achieve the same in vitro antibacterial effects.

The world's scientific literature contains hundreds of articles that validate the therapeutic use of honey for skin infections, wounds, burns, traumatic amputations, plus many hundreds more of anecdotal references to the use of honey for many diseases and conditions. Unfortunately the "slight regard . . .

paid to the medicinal virtues of Honey" written of by Dr. Hill in 1759 continues today. Perhaps one of the reasons this is so is captured by Joe Traynor when he describes honey as "A Medicine Without A Profit."[229]

Methylglyoxal and Diabetes

It is important to make a distinction between honey varietals, their effectiveness as a topical antimicrobial and their potential effects when ingested, particularly with regard to honey varietals that contain a high level of methylglyoxal. As stated above, Manuka honey which is noted for its powerful antibiotic activity, may contain up to 1000 times the amount of MGO as other non-Manuka honey. This is a critical distinction as MGO is highly cytotoxic within the human system.

Because MGO is so toxic to cells, rapid detoxification in the body is necessary. Detoxification of MGO is accomplished by a process known as non-enzymatic glycosylation. This process produces advanced glycation end-products (AGEs),[230] the same metabolites that are produced from intracellular oxidative stress due to hyperglycemia in patients with diabetes. AGEs, when attached to receptors found on cells from the lung, liver, kidney or blood, contribute to age- and diabetes-related chronic inflammatory diseases such as atherosclerosis, asthma, arthritis, myocardial infarction, kidney disease, retinopathy, and other conditions of the nervous system.[231, 232, 233]

Findings of research published in 2006, indicate that MGO is also associated with the early phases of insulin resistance. Even short exposures to MGO can lead to an inhibition of insulin-induced signaling. Thus, "methylglyoxal may not only induce the debilitating complications of diabetes but may also contribute to the pathophysiology of diabetes in general."[234] In other words, MGO not only contributes to increased oxidative stress within the cells by its rapid metabolism into AGEs, but also may be one of the causative factors of the diabetes by its inhibition of insulin.

The lesson learned from this is that while all honey is good, not all honey is good for you, especially when consumed. Many honey varietals may contain some MGO, especially honey that has been heated. In fact, some European countries test honey for MGO and ban honey imports that contain it.

Fortunately, the amount of MGO is small or none in most honey varietals. Honey containing MGO such as Manuka honey that is used specifically as a topical agent for treating superficial skin infections, wounds and burns should not be consumed, especially if one is diabetic or has abnormalities with blood sugar metabolism.

Honey as an Effective Cough Suppressant

The ability of honey or honey solutions to treat the symptoms of common upper respiratory infections (URI), sooth the throat and suppress cough has been appreciated in many cultures for centuries.[235]   The World Health Organization cited honey as a potential treatment for URI in an official publication in 2001.[236] However, it was not until 2007 that research at a reputable university medical center confirmed this finding in a clinical study involving 105 pediatric patients.

In a well-controlled, double-blinded study conducted by Dr. Ian Paul and his associates at the Penn State University College of Medicine, honey was found to be most effective in reducing cough severity and frequency in young children and in improving both child and parent sleep quality when compared to dextromethorphan (DM), the most common over-the-counter antitussive. Noting the antioxidant and antimicrobial effects of honey as possible mechanisms, the study concludes that honey "may be a preferable treatment for the cough and sleep difficulty associated with childhood upper respiratory tract infection."[237]

Common buckwheat honey, a darker honey varietal was used exclusively in the study. Buckwheat honey as well as other darker honeys is known to have higher levels of antioxidants and other phenolic compounds.

10 Honey - Nature's Miraculous Food

Chapter Summary

The processing of honey varies widely among honey producers. Understanding how honey is collected, processed and packed will help you determine which honey is best for you and your family.

Honey is packed and sold under a variety of labels. Understanding these terms becomes your guide to making informed choices. The health benefits of honey vary depending on the specific varietal so it is important to choose wisely.

Only pure, unadulterated honey will provide you with optimum health benefits.

Honey is nature's miraculous food!

If you are just discovering honey or starting to use it for health reasons, you may be a bit curious about the varieties and brands of honey available in the market. Which honey is best? What kind of honey provides the most health benefits? Is there an advantage to "local honey?"

To answer these questions, it is necessary to provide a brief description of the way honey is processed and to define a few terms that describe honey as it is sold or available today.

Honey Processing

The process of extracting honey from the hive and packing it in containers varies widely among honey producers. The hobbyist beekeeper who maintains only a few hives may extract honey manually, removing the frames of comb from the hive, shaving off the wax caps, and spinning out the honey in a small hand operated extractor (a centrifuge that rotates the frames and

147

spins out the honey). The honey is collected in buckets and it may be run through a fine pore sieve or metal filter to remove large particles, wax, and other material that has found its way into the honey during its removal from the frames. Sometimes the honey is warmed slightly to liquefy it and make the process of filing small containers easier.

Commercial honey producers may keep several hundred to several thousand hives. Honey extraction for the commercial producer is highly mechanized. Hives are collected from multiple bee yards and brought to an extracting facility or "honey house." Frames are removed from the hives by mechanized automated processors that uncap the comb, place the frames in giant extractors and spin out the honey. Honey is collected, run through a sieve and pumped into large tanks which hold the honey until it is pumped into 55 gallon drums, sealed and stored until sold or needed for the next step in processing. Depending on the temperature and length of time kept in the drums until the honey is processed and packed, the honey will crystallize and become quite solid. Honey will keep indefinitely in sealed drums and will not spoil. Some commercial honey producers maintain millions of pounds of honey in storage from year to year.

Honey Terms

Honey is packaged and sold under a host of labels using various terms that are not well defined. The following definitions of terms are offered to provide the honey buyer information on which to make advised decisions rather than to indicate the advantages of one over the other.

Raw honey is honey that has not been heated or combined with diatomaceous earth and filtered through a micro-pore filter. Raw honey is pure honey. Nothing has been added or removed.

Comb Honey is honey that is packed with a portion of the comb included. The wax comb from the frame in the hive is cut into pieces and packed into tubs or jars with honey. This process "destroys" the comb making this method of selling honey much more expensive as the comb is not available for reuse. Some comb honey is actually produced directly by the honeybees in the small 6 or 8 ounce tub-sized portions in which it is sold. The small empty containers are placed in the hive within a frame. Honeybees create new comb within the small tubs and fill it with honey. This method of producing comb honey is nature's way of automating production! Many folks prefer comb honey and use it as a spread, wax and all, for toast.

Granulated or crystallized honey is honey in which the sugars have become crystallized naturally over time. All honey will crystallize eventually given normal conditions. The honey becomes thick, almost solid. This honey has not turned bad and need not be discarded. Simply place the honey container in a warm water bath not exceeding 110 degrees F for a period of time until the honey returns to its liquid state.

Spun honey or creamed honey as it is sometimes called is honey that has been artificially crystallized and spun or whipped until reaching a uniform spreadable consistency. The processing of spun honey requires that liquid honey first be heated to dissolve any larger crystals that may be in the honey. Then smaller seed crystals are added to the honey and the honey is spun or whipped until the honey is crystalized evenly throughout the batch. Fruit or other flavors may be added to the honey to produce flavored spun honey. The pre-crystallized honey is then placed in plastic or glass containers and labeled for resale.

In Europe, spun honey is preferred by much of the honey consuming public. The shelf live is longer since the honey will not crystallize further and if kept in a cooler environment, the honey will not liquefy.

Blended honey refers to honey from multiple sources that has been mixed together prior to bottling or packing. Blended honey may come from several domestic sources or imported from various countries. It is not yet required on labels to indicate that honey has been blended from multiple sources. Neither is there a labeling requirement in the United States that requires a "Country of Origin" statement on the label. Hence, honey that is packed or bottled by several of the large honey packing companies and resold as generic US Grade A Honey may be honey from many sources.

Pure honey is simply that - natural honey with nothing added. However, it is not the intent of this book to perpetuate the myth that honey dwells in a realm of ultra purity. All "pure honey" will contain trace amounts of foreign substances and/or contaminants. These trace substances may include residues of pesticides, antibiotics, anti-mite chemicals or other substances that the honeybee may come into contact with while gathering nectar and pollen. As there currently are no requirements for testing for contaminants in honey in the U.S., information regarding trace amounts of these substances that may or may not be found in honey are not readily available.

Organic honey may be purchased in the United States but most, if not all of it, is imported honey. Honeybees will fly up to three miles to gather nectar and there are few areas in the U.S. where nectar producing blossoms exist that are not exposed to agricultural or industrial chemicals. Organic honey is available from Brazil. However when purchasing organic honey, one must keep in mind that the certification processes for organic foods may differ from country to country.

U.S. Grade A Honey is found on the labels of many honey brands and varietals. This label is somewhat misleading as there are no grading **requirements** for honey packed or sold in the U.S. Grading Standards do exist and have been published by the USDA, however they are voluntary standards and serve as a basis for inspection and grading by the Federal inspection service. A copy of the Extracted Honey Standards and the grading criteria is included in Appendix B.

Heating honey is required in the packing or bottling of honey to decrease its viscosity and allow it to pass through filters or sieves to remove contaminants. Most honey packers heat honey from 140 to 160 degrees F to dissolve any crystals and lengthen its shelf life. Heating honey above 160 degrees for a lengthy period of time will change the character and color of honey. Heating honey also increases the amount of methylglyoxal (MGO) that it contains. Heating honey may kill some of the heat-labile enzymes contained in honey.

Strained honey refers to honey that has been run through a fine pore metal sieve to remove wax or other particulate matter that may be present. Strained honey is an official type of extracted honey as defined in the USDA Grading Standards. There is no component for clarity for strained honey as there is for filtered honey.

Filtered honey is also an official type of extracted honey as defined by the USDA Grading Standards. The process of filtering honey is facilitated by the addition of diatomaceous earth (DE), a process used by most large honey packers. Diatomaceous earth consists of fossilized remains of a type of hard-shelled algae (diatoms). The powdery DE acts as an absorbent removing ultra fine particles that may be found in the honey. The process involves adding DE to the honey, heating it and then filtering the honey through a series of fine micro-filters to remove all micro-contaminants including most of the DE. Much of the beneficial pollen residues naturally contained in honey is also removed by filtering with DE.

Most small honey packers or honey producers that pack their own honey for resale at farmer's markets do not filter honey. Frequently one will see "unfiltered" on the label on honey sold in retail stores to indicate that the honey has only been strained and not filtered with DE before it has been packed. Unfiltered honey will crystallize or granulate sooner than DE filtered honey. If this happens, simply heat the honey container in a warm water bath (110 degrees) until it returns to a liquid state. It is not recommended that a microwave be used to heat honey.

Tolerance Limits for Contaminants in Honey

Honeybees are fragile insects. It is the responsibility of the beekeeper to tend his bees in such a way as to promote their healthy state. Throughout the year, honeybees will need treatment with chemicals to prevent mite infestations. Antibiotics may need to be applied in the hive for bacterial infections that can destroy a hive. Trace levels of these chemicals and antibiotics may be present in honey. Most of these are not harmful to humans at the levels (usually in fractions of a part per million) found in honey.

These trace levels need not unnecessarily concern honey consumers for this reason. The amount of honey consumed daily is typically a very small amount. Even when ingested in the amounts suggested in parts of this book, the daily or even yearly dose of honey consumed is not such that trace contaminants would cause harm to an individual.

In the European Union where there are harmonized laws defining tolerance limits of residues in foods including honey, the situation approaches the absurd. For example, residues of non-banned antibiotics <1 part per billion (ppb) are frequently objected to and published in the rapid alert system for foods, depending on the political interest and scope. Everyone recognizes that insistence on absolute tolerance limits is nonsensical but politicians primarily follow their national interests instead of finding an acceptable compromise.

These above statements are not meant to excuse or rationalize the presence of trace contaminants in honey. Rather they are meant to encourage the adoption of reasonable tolerance limits based on good science. For a list of EPA tolerance levels or Minimum Residual Levels for chemicals in honey and other agricultural commodities, see Appendix C.

Honey Varietals

Honey, like wine, can be purchased in multiple floral and taste variations. Most of the honey consumed in the US is from a combination of several unidentified floral nectar sources. This honey is commonly labeled as "clover honey" and may contain honey from other floral nectars. This is typically a blended honey described above.

When one ventures away from the routine and begins to try different honey varietals, one quickly discovers the amazing qualities and taste sensations of various honeys. It may be necessary for one to visit a health food store or specialty kitchen shop to find these varietals, but the effort will be worth it. One will discover personal favorites, like orange blossom honey, lavender honey, eucalyptus honey or even wild flower honey from the western slopes of Colorado.

By the same process, one will discover honey varietals that are destined to sit untouched on the pantry shelf to crystallize. An example that comes to mind in this category is raw unfiltered coffee flower honey from the highlands of Chiapas, Mexico. Tastes like the worst medicine! Perhaps it is very good for you.

Honey Varietals and Health Benefits

A honey varietal will make a difference as to the health benefit it offers. We have mentioned in Chapter 9 above that Manuka honey is a particular varietal that possesses powerful antibiotic characteristics. However, the methylglyoxal content of Manuka honey renders it particularly dangerous for individuals with diabetes or glucose intolerance.

Leptospermum honey is honey made from the flower of the leptospermum tree found in New Zealand and Australia. Leptospermum honey or Manuka honey as it is known in New Zealand is the primary ingredient used in **MediHoney™** Active Leptospermum Honey dressings available in the UK and Europe, Australia and the United States. **MediHoney™** is also available in sterilized tubes and jars.

Darker honeys have been found to possess higher concentrations of antioxidants which afford many healthful benefits. Buckwheat honey, as described in Chapter 9 works as an inexpensive and efficient cough suppressant. Beyond this there are a whole host of heath benefits that are provided from most honey varietals.

Additional research is underway in Canada, Europe, and New Zealand to document the health benefits of many honey varietals, their active ingredients, and the physiologic mechanisms by which they work within the human system. As more research is completed, we may find that other varieties of honey have specific health benefits.

The Great American Honey Heist

A darker side of the American honey industry exists and must be told. Passing references to honey purity and adulteration of honey can be found in the above narrative. Here we will present more of the story providing a glimpse of the fraud and deception that has plagued the world honey industry for several years.

In 2007 U.S. honey producers accounted for approximately 150 million pounds of the nearly 360 million pounds of honey consumed. That means that approximately sixty percent of the honey consumed in the United States was imported. As there are no testing requirements or standards for honey except on a voluntary basis, much of the honey that has been imported into the U.S. is not honey at all but a diluted or adulterated product made of corn syrup or corn syrup and honey blends. Corn syrup is much cheaper to produce than honey. It is relatively easy to flavor corn syrup and/or to mix it with pure honey to create an imitation substance that looks like honey and tastes like honey but is not honey. Check the fine print on a small packet of "honey" provided with the hot biscuit at KFC the next time you have the opportunity.

The drivers for this unfortunate situation are economics and greed. The Chinese have been implicit in this for several years. In 2007, antidumping laws were passed and huge tariffs were imposed on Chinese honey imports to correct the problem. In January 2008, imports of Chinese honey were reduced to only five percent of what they had been a year before. The few containers of Chinese honey that did enter the U.S. had values in the range of only $0.09 to 0.12 per pound as compared to the then current market value of nearly $1.00 per pound.

However shortly after the enactment of corrective tariffs in 2007 a new problem emerged. Honey began arriving in the United States from countries that historically were minor producers of honey or from countries that had not previously been honey exporters. Some honey shipments even arrived with documents indicating that the honey came from Russia and other countries which could not account for this honey ever having been in those countries. Not only was imported honey arriving as a diluted or adulterated product, its shipments were being circumvented through countries that produce very little or no honey to avoid tariffs.

Several unscrupulous companies both here and abroad have been complicit in this fraud. Most of these have established relationships with overseas Chinese business interests. In May 2008 arrests of company executives of a major food import company in Chicago were announced. Officers of another firm in Texas were indicted. A major customs investigation began to uncover and unravel the fraud and deception.

For many American honey producers, this correction will come too late. Many have closed up their facilities or sold out to larger producers. Fortunately, the price of honey began to rise during the early part of 2008. But this too is a bitter sweet pill. With the value of the U.S. dollar falling to low levels, honey imports into the country must compete with countries paying with the much stronger Euro. Major honey exporters from Brazil and Argentina, Uruguay and Chile look to Europe as their preferred market.

Couple this with the continuing crisis of what is referred to as Colony Collapse Disorder or CCD which has been resulting in annual losses of between thirty to forty percent of existing colonies, the U.S. beekeeper faces a challenging near future. The one bright spot is that honey prices continue to rise forestalling economic disaster for many beekeepers. Given improved economic incentives and market corrections destined to occur worldwide, there is light at the end of the tunnel.

There is Nothing New Under the Sun

One fascinating historical note illustrates that adulteration of honey is not a new problem. In 1878, a petition was drawn up by Charles Dadant and sent to the Congress of the United States, signed by more than 30,000 individuals. The petition content is reproduced on page 156 as published in Eva Crane's book, **Honey A Comprehensive Survey**.[238]

The unfortunate fact remains that as of the date of publication of this book, only one state (Florida) has enacted what is known as "Standard of Identity" laws defining honey. While many countries in the world have quality standards for honey, the United States does not.

Final Thoughts

There are important messages for the honey consumer in all of this that must not be overlooked. Honey is a natural product whose identity and purity must be protected, celebrated and appreciated. In the absence of mandatory standards and regulations, the best recourse for the consumer is to buy honey from local producers whose name and reputation depends on producing a quality product. Be conscious of price. When one can buy honey in the big box stores at a price of less per pound than it takes to produce a pound of honey, it may be wise to question what it is that one is potentially buying.

When considering the healthful benefits of honey as presented in detail in this book, remember that only pure natural honey can deliver these benefits. Diluted, adulterated, or imitation products will fall short at best and at worst contribute to the multiple conditions associated with the consumption of sugar, high fructose corn syrup and other sweeteners.

As healthcare professionals and authors who have spent much time researching, writing and speaking about honey and health, it continues to be a source of amazement to witness the responses of many upon hearing just a few of the facts presented in this book. Many are simply overwhelmed by the volume of factual information that attributes to honey the many healthful benefits that it possesses. Others find the often counter-intuitive logic of honey's health message to be refreshing, even revolutionary. Most immediately relate some symptom or another that they have been struggling with for months or years for which honey offers relief. A few are skeptical.

Were it not for extensive contemporary validation for the many health benefits of honey found in the world's scientific literature, some of what has been presented in this book would simply sound preposterous. Though some findings are preliminary, there is sufficient indication from research conducted within the past five years to differentiate honey from other sweeteners. Honey is in a class of its own when it comes to liver metabolism and glycogen storage. Honey's ability to control or eliminate metabolic stress and thereby reduce the risk for many diseases borders on miraculous. Honey's role as an effective antimicrobial is just beginning to be appreciated in the western world.

Honey is a revolutionary natural food!

Consider the following statements that summarize the rather amazing benefits of consuming pure natural honey:

- *Honey is a preferred sweetener for diabetics* as regular consumption **lowers** blood sugar levels.
- *Honey fuels the liver and the brain* by facilitating glycogen formation and storage.

- *Honey reduces metabolic stress* reducing the risks for insulin resistance, diabetes, and the conditions related to the metabolic syndrome.
- *Regular honey consumption will result in weight loss* and reduced percentage of body fat.
- *Honey facilitates and promotes restorative sleep and recovery physiology.*
- *Honey reduces the risk of cardiovascular disease and hypertension.*
- *Honey consumption will result in lower cholesterol, lower triglycerides, and increases in HDL-cholesterol.*
- *Honey improves and restores the immune system.*
- *Honey improves memory*, creative thought, and off-line processing.
- *Honey consumption reduces anxiety and helps alleviate depression.*
- *Honey reduces oxidative stress within neural (brain) tissue* resulting in reductions in the risk for Alzheimer's Disease, dementia and other neuro-degenerative diseases.
- *Honey reduces risks for certain forms of cancers.*
- *Honey will reduce gum and periodontal disease* by its powerful antibiotic activity.
- *Honey combats many gastrointestinal disorders* and works as a powerful probiotic within the GI tract.
- *Honey is a most effective cough suppressant.*

The regular consumption of from three to five tablespoons per day of natural unfiltered honey does all of this and more without side effects, risks or negative health consequences.

For your good health, join the Honey Revolution.

Petition to the United States Senate and Congress, 1878

> **To the Honorable Senate and House of Representatives of the United States:**
>
> Your Petitioners respectfully represent to your honorable body: -
>
> 1. That the sweets now in use in the United States, including cane-sugar, maple-sugar, syrups, candies, jellies, *honey* (emphasis added), etc., are often adulterated with glucose, and sometimes are manufactured entirely of it.
>
> 2. That this glucose is manufactured from corn starch, by boiling the starch with sulphuric acid, (oil of vitriol), then mixing it with lime. The glucose always retains more or less of sulphuric acid and lime, and sometimes it has copperas, sucrate of lime, etc.
>
> 3. That seventeen specimens of common table syrups, were recently examined by R.C. Kedzie, A.M., Professor of Chemistry in the Michigan State Agricultural College, at Lansing. Fifteen of these proved to be made of glucose; one of the fifteen contained 141 grains of sulphuric acid, (oil of vitriol), and 724 grains of lime to the gallon; and another which had caused serious sickness in a whole family, contained 72 grains of sulphuric acid, 28 grains of sulphate of iron, (copperas), and 363 grains of lime to the gallon.
>
> 4. That the American people are pre-eminently a sugar-eating people. The consumption of sugar, by each individual in our country, is shown by statistics to be about 40 pounds a year. It is seen at once that the adulterators of sugars and other sweets, not only cheat our people in the quality of what they consume, since glucose contains only from 30 to 40 percent of sugar, but injure also the public health, by selling under false names, an article injurious to health.
>
> 5. It is as much the right and duty of Congress to enact laws against such frauds in food as it is to enact laws against frauds in money, for if the counterfeiters of money injure the public wealth, the counterfeiters of food injure the public health.
>
> In view of the above facts your petitioners earnestly request your honorable body to decree that the adulteration of sweets, and the sale of such adulterated products, are crimes against the people, and to enact laws for the suppression of this illegal business.
>
> And your petitioners will ever pray.

Appendix A - Composition of Honey

In addition to the typical components of honey as listed in the table on page 23, the following substances (some found in very small trace amounts) are known to be found in natural honey:

Acids found in honey:
Acetic
Butyric
Citric
Formic
Gluconic
Lactic
Maleic
Malic
Oxalic
Pyroglutamic
Succinic
Glycollic
a-ketoglutaric
Pyruvic
Tartaric
2- or 3-phosphoglyceric
a- or B-glycerophosphate
Glucose-6-phosphate

Amino Acids in honey:
Lysine
Histidine
Arginine
Aspartic acid
Threonine
Serine
Glutamic acid
Proline
Glycine
Alanine
Cystine
Valine
Methionine
*Iso*leucine
Leucine
Tyrosine
Tryptophan
Phenylalanine

Minerals in honey:
Potassium
Sodium
Calcium
Calcium as lime
Magnesium
Iron
Copper
Manganese
Chlorine
Phosphorus
Sulphur
Silica

Enzymes in honey:
Diastase
Invertase
Glucose oxidase
Catalase
Acid Phosphatase

Aroma Constituents in honey:
Carbonyls (9)
Alcohols (14)
Esters (3)

Trace Elements in honey:
Chromium
Lithium
Nickel
Lead
Tin
Zinc
Osmium
Beryllium
Vanadium
Zirconium
Silver
Barium
Gallium
Bismuth
Gold
Germanium
Strontium

Vitamins in honey:
Riboflavin
Pantothenic acid
Niacin
Thiamine
Pyridoxine
Ascorbic acid

Lipids:

Phospholipids
Glycerides
Sterols
Oleic Acid
Linoleic acid
Lauric acid
Myristoleic acid
Stearric acid

In all there are over 180 substances known to be present in honey. The above list is taken from: "Honey - A Comprehensive Survey," Edited by Eva Crane, Crane, Russak & Company, Inc. (1975)

Appendix B - Natural and Artificial Sugar Substitutes

The three primary compounds used as sugar substitutes in the United States are saccharin (e.g., Sweet'N Low), aspartame (e.g., Equal, NutraSweet) and sucralose (e.g., Splenda). In many other countries cyclamate and the herbal sweetener stevia are used extensively.

Natural Sugar Substitutes	Type of Compound	Sweetness compared to Sucrose (by weight)
Brazzein	Protein	800 X
Curulin	Protein	550 X
Erythritol	Sugar Alcohol	0.7 X (14 X by food energy)
Fructose	Sugar	1.7 X
Glycyrrhizin	Liquorice root extract	30-50 X
Glycerol	Sugar Alcohol	0.6 X (0.55 X by food energy)
Lactitol	Sugar Alcohol	0.4 X
Lo Han Guo	Fruit extract	300 X
Mabinlin	Protein	100 X
Maltitol	Sugar Alcohol	0.9 X (1.7 X by food energy)
Mannitol	Sugar Alcohol	0.5 X (1.2 X by food energy)
Miraculin	Protein	Does not taste sweet
Monellin	Protein	3000 X
Pentadin	Protein	500 X

Sorbitol	Sugar Alcohol	0.6 X (0.9 X by food energy)
Stevia	Plant extract	250 X
Tagatose	A monosaccharide from dairy products	0.92 X (2.4 X by food energy)
Thaumatin	Protein	200 X
Xylitol	Sugar Alcohol	1.0 X (1.7 X by food energy)
Artificial Sugar Substitutes	**Trade or Brand Name**	**Sweetness compared to Sucrose (by weight)**
Acesulfame potassium	Nutrinova	200 X
Alitame		2000 X
Aspartame	NutraSweet	160-200 X
Salt of aspartame-acelulfame	Twinsweet	350 X
Cyclamate		30 X
Dulcin		250 X
Glucin		300 X
Neohesperidin dihydrochalcone		1500 X
Neatame	NutraSweet	8000 X
P-4000		4000 X
Saccharin		300 X
Sucralose	Splenda	600 X
Isomalt		0.45-0.65 X (0.9-1.3 X by food energy)

[The information above is from Wikipedia - section entitled "Sugar Substitute"]

[Note: several of the sugar substitutes listed in the tables above are not available in the United States having been banned by the FDA. Some are still undergoing evaluation and have not been released for use in the U.S.]

Appendix C - Extracted Honey Standards

Is the honey you pack or consume U.S. Grade A, B, C or substandard? This is not a rhetorical question. The above grades exist and are published in the fifth issue, as amended, of the United States Standards for Grades of Extracted Honey published in the Federal Register of April 23, 1985 (50 FR 15861) to become effective May 23, 1985. This supercedes the fourth issue, in effect since April 16, 1951.

Standards are set by a cumulative number of points based on several factors. Color (water white to dark amber) is not used in grading. Two official types of extracted honey exist, *filtered* and *strained*. The filtered contains a component for clarity, the strained does not; everything else remains the same for both types.

Two kinds of factors exist to grade honey: analytical (use of an instrument like a refractometer to determine soluble solids), an objective test, and quality (absence of defects, flavor and aroma, clarity), subjective at best. The following is an abbreviated chart to determine grades:

FACTORS	Grade A	Grade B	Grade C	Substandard
% Soluble Solids	81.4	81.4	80	Fails Grade C
Absence of Defects	Practically free	Reasonably Free	Fairly Free	Fails Grade C
Score Points	37-40	34-36	31-33	0-30
Flavor & Aroma	Good	Reasonably Good	Fairly Good	Fails Grade C
Score Points	45-50	40-44	35-39	0-34
Clarity	Clear	Reasonably Clear	Fairly Clear	Fails Grade C
Score Points	8 - 10	6 - 7	4 - 5	0 - 3
Total Minimum Score Points	90	80	70	Fails Grade C

Notice that percent solids of 81.4 means a moisture content of 18.6. Also if absence of defects or flavor and aroma fall into the substandard category, they cannot be graded any higher regardless of total score.

Those classed as filtered honey and falling into the substandard area with respect to clarity cannot be graded above grade C regardless of total score. Categorizing such samples as strained, however, will get around this problem.

At present the standards are voluntary and available for use by producers, suppliers, buyers and consumers. They also serve as a basis for inspection and grading by the Federal inspection service, the ONLY ACTIVITY AUTHORIZED TO APPROVE the designation of U.S. grades as referenced in the standards. This service is available as on-line (in-plant) or lot inspection and grading of all processed fruit and vegetable products on a fee basis. For more information and to receive a copy of the standards, write the Chief, Processed Products Branch, Fruit and Vegetable Division, AMS, USDA, Washington, D.C. 20250.

Appendix D - EPA Absolute Tolerance Levels / Minimum Residual Levels for Honey

Chemical	Trade Name	EPA Tolerance in Parts Per Million / Parts Per Billion (ppm/ppb)
Coumaphos	Check-mite	0.10 ppm / 100 ppb
Fluvalinate	Apistan	0.05 ppm / 50 ppb
Tylosin	Tylan	0.20 ppm / 200 ppb *
Oxytetracycline	Terramycin	0.01 ppm / 10 ppb **

*No EPA tolerance level. This is based on maximum residues. The maximum residue of 200 ppb also applies to many other agricultural commodities (chick, turkey, cattle, swine, eggs).

** Limit of detection should not be measurable if label directions for usage are followed.

Appendix E - Posters

Reproductions of the posters which follow were prepared for and first presented at the First International Symposium on Honey and Human Health held in Sacramento, California on January 8, 2008. There are included here as a complete set and reproduced with the permission of the Committee for the Promotion of Honey and Health, Inc. Full color copies of these posters are available at *www.prohoneyandhealth.com*.

Index of Posters

INTRODUCTION TO POSTER SESSION

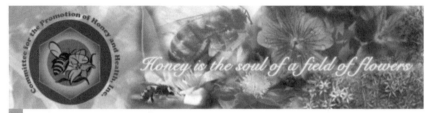

[These posters were first presented at the First International Symposium on Honey and Human Health held in Sacramento, CA on January 8, 2008]

INTRODUCTION TO POSTER SESSION

The Committee for the Promotion of Health and Honey, Inc is pleased to present the following series of numbered posters for your information and education. The posters are based on research or original articles previously published from the world's scientific literature. The careful reader will note that not all of the posters have a direct or obvious relationship to the consumption of honey. This is a critical fact not meant to confuse the reader. Some of these posters provide important foundational information upon which the health implications of honey, when consumed regularly, are based. The reader is guided by the comments provided by the editors which underscore these implications. Thank you for taking the time to view these posters. We respect and appreciate your comments and questions.

NOTE: Additional posters that are not part of this numbered series 1-16 are from presentations given at the First International Symposium on Honey and Human Health and contain information from previously published works. These posters have been prepared by the authors and/or the speakers themselves. References to these posters or their content in any media or reproductions must contain appropriate citations.

© Mike McInnes, MRPS and Ronald E Fessenden, MD, MPH, December 2007

The Committee for the Promotion of Honey and Health, Inc

www.prohoneyandhealth.com

For additional information please contact

info@prohoneyandhealth.com

720-851-0386 (Office Phone)

303-840-7251 (Fax)

Appendix E

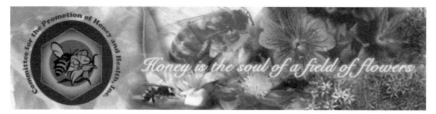

POSTER NO 1

The Effect of Honey on Prostaglandin Levels in the Body

Al-Waili, Noori S, M.D, PhD; and BONI, NADER S, M.Sc; "Natural Honey Lowers Plasma Prostaglandin Concentrations in Normal Individuals", **Journal of Medicinal Food**, 2003 Summer; 6 (2): 129-33

ABSTRACT

Twelve normal, healthy adult individuals, 9 men and 3 women, 25–48 years of age (mean, 38 years), were recruited in the study. After 12 hours of fasting, blood specimens were collected at 8:00 AM for prostaglandin E2 (PGE2), PGF2a, and thromboxane B2 assays. Each individual then drank 250 ml of water containing 1.2 g/kg body weight of natural unprocessed honey, after which collection of blood was repeated at 1, 2, and 3 hours for estimation of prostaglandins. Each individual was asked to drink the same amount of honey diluted in water once a day for a maximum of 15 days. After 12 hours of fasting, morning blood specimens were collected on day 16, and plasma prostaglandin concentrations were measured. The quantitative analysis of prostaglandins was performed with use of an enzyme-linked immunosorbent (ELISA) test. Results showed that the mean plasma concentration of thromboxane B2 was reduced by 7%, 34%, and 35%, and that of PGE2 by 14%, 10%, and 19%, at 1, 2, and 3 hours, respectively, after honey ingestion. The level of PGF2a was decreased by 31% at 2 hours and 14% at 3 hours after honey ingestion. At day 15, plasma concentrations of thromboxane B2, PGE2, and PGF2a were decreased by 48%, 63%, and 50%, respectively. It may be concluded that honey can lower the concentrations of prostaglandins in plasma of normal individuals.

COMMENT

Prostaglandins, in the human system, are potent "mediators" of a variety of strong physiological effects. They are technically hormones, although they are rarely classified as such. The prostaglandins together with the thromboxanes form a class of fatty acid derivatives.

There are nine known prostaglandin receptors on various cell types in the body. These varied receptors mean that prostaglandins act on a variety of cells, and have a wide variety of actions. Prostaglandins:

- cause constriction or dilatation in vascular smooth muscle cells
- cause aggregation or dis-aggregation of platelets
- sensitize spinal neurons to pain
- constrict smooth muscle
- regulate inflammatory mediation
- regulate calcium movement
- regulate hormone regulation
- control cell growth

In general, prostaglandins are thought of as mediators of inflammation in the body. Both prostaglandins and thromboxanes have been implicated in immune suppression and atherosclerosis.

This small and limited study demonstrates that honey may lower prostaglandin levels in normal individuals. To the degree that honey lowers prostaglandin levels, it may be considered to have an anti-inflammatory effect in the body.

Additional References:
1. Kozlov V, Poveschenko A, Gromyhina N, "Some mechanism involved in the prostaglandin E2 immunosuppressive effect in F1 mice in vivo". **Cellular Immunology** 1990;128:242–249.
2. Colina-Chourio A, Gody-Gody N and Avila-Hernandez R M, "Role of prostaglandins in hypertension" **Journal of Human Hypertension** April 2000 Vol 14, ppS16-S193
3. Robertson Pr, Chein Mei, "Role of Prostagladin E in Defective Insulin Secretion and Carbohydrate Intolerance in Diabetes Mellitus". **Journal of Clinical Investigation** 1977 60(3): 747-753

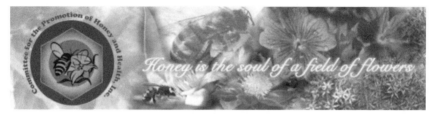

POSTER NO 2

Honey Protects against the Hypertriglyceridemic effect of Fructose

Busserolles, Jérôme; Gueux, Elyett; Rock, Edmond; Mazur, Andrzej and Rayssiguier, Yves; "Substituting Honey for Refined Carbohydrates Protects Rats from Hypertriglyceridemic and Prooxidative Effects of Fructose", **American Society of Nutritional Sciences Journal of Nutrition,** 132:3370-3382 Nov 2002.

Recent findings indicate that a high fructose diet has a pro-oxidant effect in rats compared with a starch diet. Because honey is rich in fructose, the aim of this study was to assess the effect of substituting honey for refined carbohydrates on lipid metabolism and oxidative stress. Rats were fed for 2 weeks purified diets containing 65 g/100 g carbohydrates as wheat starch or a combination of fructose and glucose or a honey-based diet prepared by substituting honey for refined carbohydrates (n = 9/group). The same amount of fructose was provided by the honey and fructose diets. The hypertriglyceridemic effect of fructose was not observed when fructose was provided by honey. Compared with those fed starch, fructose-fed rats had a lower plasma-tocopherol level, higher plasma nitrite and nitrate (NOx) levels and were less protected from lipid peroxidation as indicated by heart homogenate TBARS concentration. Compared with those fed fructose, honey-fed rats had a higher plasma-tocopherol level, a higher ocopherol/triacylglycerol ratio, lower plasma NOx concentrations and a lower susceptibility of heart to lipid peroxidation. Further studies are required to identify the mechanism underlying the antioxidant effect of honey but the data suggest a potential nutritional benefit of substituting honey for fructose in the diet.

COMMENT

This animal study above demolishes the notion that because honey contains fructose, it must therefore express the pro-oxidative effect and result in elevated circulating triglyceride levels as known to occur with a diet high in fructose (as in high fructose corn syrup or HFCS). Honey-fed rats showed lower levels of triglycerides and lowered pro-oxidant effects than those fed starch or HFCS. Additional human studies are required to identify mechanisms responsible for this effect.

Another study to be presented at this Symposium will confirm these results and further indicate that honey diets are preferable to refined sugar or HFCS diets with regard to weight gain, HA1c and triglyceride levels.

Additional Referrences:

1. Busseroles J, Rock E, Gueux E, Mazur A, Rayssiguier Y. "Short-term consumption of a high-sucrose diet has a pro-oxidant effect in rats".
2. Elliott, Sharon S; Keim, Nancy L; Stern, Judith S; Teff, Karen; and Peter J; "Fructose, weight gain and the insulin resistance syndrome". **Journal of Nutrition,** Apr,87 (4): 337-4

Appendix E

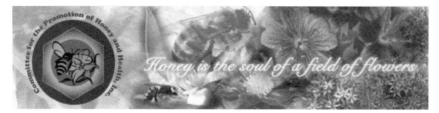

POSTER NO 3

Metabolic Risk for Diabetes with Short and Long Sleep

H. Klar Yaggi, MD, MPH, Andre B. Araujo, PHD and John B. McKinlay, PHD, "Sleep Duration as a Risk Factor for the Development of Type 2 Diabetes", **Diabetes Care** 29:657-661, 2006

OBJECTIVE

Short-term partial sleep restriction results in glucose intolerance and insulin resistance. The purpose of this study was to assess the long-term relationship between sleep duration and the incidence of clinical diabetes.

RESULTS

Men reporting short sleep duration (5 and 6 hours of sleep per night) were twice as likely to develop diabetes, and men reporting long sleep duration (> 8 hours of sleep per night) were more than three times as likely to develop diabetes over the period of follow-up. Elevated risks remained essentially unchanged after adjustment for age, hypertension, smoking status, self-rated health status, education, and waist circumference (RR 1.95 [95% CI 0.95–4.01] for 5 hours and 3.12 [1.53–6.37] for >8 hours). Relative Risks were altered considerably for the two extreme sleep groups when adjusted for testosterone (1.51 [0.71–3.19] for 5 hours and 2.81 [1.34–5.90] for > 8 hours), suggesting that the effects of sleep on diabetes could be mediated via changes in endogenous testosterone levels.

CONCLUSIONS

Short and long sleep durations increase the risk of developing diabetes, independent of confounding factors. Sleep duration may represent a novel risk factor for diabetes.

COMMENT

This observational study points up the relationship between both short and long sleep to diabetes. Within the context of liver glycogen plenitude during the night fast, we have an explanation as to why more than 8 hours of sleep, with increased release of adrenal stress hormones, contributes to an increased risk of diabetes. Liver glycogen depletion during long rest periods contributes to the release of those hormones and produces the associated detrimental effects. The adrenal hormone cortisol is the main hormone produced by the body that contributes to the development of insulin resistance and type II diabetes.

Replenishing the liver with honey prior to bed may reduce the release of these adrenal stress hormones overnight and thus diminish the risk for insulin resistance and type II diabetes.

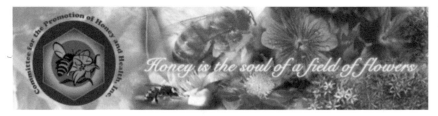

POSTER NO 4

Honey Protects Against Homocysteine Elevation in Rats

El-Saleh, Saleh C, "Vascular Disease Prevention", Volume 3, Number 4, November 2006 , pp. 313-318(6)

ABSTRACT

Elevated levels of plasma homocysteine (Hcy), known as hyperhomocysteinemia (HHcy), appear to be associated with higher risks of occlusive vascular disease and various clinical conditions ranging from the fetus to the elderly and from cardiovascular and neuro-degenerative diseases to neuropsychiatric disorders, rheumatoid arthritis and osteoporosis. The exact mechanism(s) involved is not fully understood. Current interest is focused upon modulating the levels of Hcy and/or their negative impacts through natural preventive strategies. In this regard, we recently showed that the Black seed (Nigella sativa), its oil, and its active ingredient Thymoquinone impart high protection (72-100%) against the induced rise of HHcy in rats.

In this investigation, the ability of natural honey to protect against HHcy in rats was investigated. The results show that honey administered to rats at 1% in water significantly improved growth and imparted a protective effect against HHcy (54.5 ± 8.0%) induced by feeding the animals a diet enriched in methionine and deficient in B-vitamins (M+B- diet) for two months. This protection was not accompanied by a decrease in concentration of ADMA (asymmetrical dimethylarginine), which may indicate that ADMA concentrations may not be related to the pathophysiology of HHcy. On the other hand, HHcy induced a 30.7 ± 0.8% drop in the antioxidant enzyme superoxidase dismutase (SOD) activity. Honey treatment recovered an 8.8 ± 1.7 % of the decrease in SOD activity. Furthermore, treatment with honey in the HHcy state decreased catalase antioxidant activity by 47.8 ± 3.9%, while it did not cause any effect on the honey-treated control rats fed a standard methionine and B-vitamin diet, indicating that honey which can release H2O2 can compromise the H2O2-neutralizing activity of the catalase enzyme under excess methionine and deficient B-vitamin conditions. Honey treatment on the other hand, did not significantly affect glutathione peroxidase activity and total antioxidant status in the control and the M+B--fed rats, while in the same rats it significantly increased the antioxidant agent uric acid by 41.5 ± 3.0 % and 33.4 ± 2.0 %, respectively. These results indicate an overall beneficial role of honey under conditions favoring HHcy (emphasis added), and the important role of B-vitamins in the defense against oxidative parameters such as H2O2 and superoxide anion.

COMMENT

Elevated levels of homocysteine (Hcy), an amino acid, are associated with an increased risk of heart disease, osteoporosis and Alzheimer's disease. This animal study demonstrates that natural honey has a significant lowering effect on homocysteine. The study results indicated that honey in only a 1% solution fed to rats improved growth, and provided protection against elevated homocysteine levels.

This is another stunning example of honey metabolism and its physiologic effects not available via the consumption of other refined sugars such as sucrose and high fructose corn syrup.

Appendix E

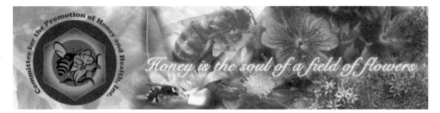

POSTER NO 5

Sleepless in America

AN EDITORIAL from the ARCHIVES OF INTERNAL MEDICINE

Joseph Bass, MD, PhD, and Fred W. Turek, MD, "Sleepless in America, A Pathway to Obesity and the Metabolic Syndrome", (REPRINTED) ARCHIVES OF INTERNAL MEDICINE, Vol. 165, January 10, 2005.

SELECTED TEXT

". . . In recent years, a new and unexpected "obesity villain" has emerged, first from laboratory studies and now, as reported by Vorona, *et al*, in this issue of the ARCHIVES, in population-based studies: insufficient sleep. In a study analyzing 924 patients from 4 primary care practices in Virginia, a reduced amount of sleep was associated with overweight and obese status, and patients in the obese group showed a near inverse linear relationship between weight and reported sleep time. The relationship between obesity (and associated metabolic and cardiovascular disorders often referred to as the metabolic syndrome, or "syndrome X") and insufficient sleep has only emerged in the past 5 years. In a pioneering study in 1999 by Van Cauter and colleagues, it was found that sleep restricted to only 4 hours per night for 1 week led to endocrine and metabolic changes associated with diabetes (insulin resistance) and weight gain in healthy young men. While the effects were reversible with normal sleep times, these remarkable, and at the time surprising findings, led basic and clinical researchers off on the trail to find the physiological linkages between insufficient sleep and metabolic function. This work also renewed interest in the role of insufficient sleep as a cause of many of the metabolic abnormalities associated with sleep apnea. However, while there is a growing awareness among some sleep, metabolic, cardiovascular, and diabetes researchers that insufficient sleep could be leading to a cascade of disorders, few in the general medical profession or in the lay public have yet made the connection. . .

An alarming statistic defines a major problem among American youth: between 1980 and 2000, the rate of obese young people has risen from 5% to 15%, and another 15% has moved into that classification in young adulthood. While this epidemic in our young population has received national attention, less well-known is the finding that children of all ages in America are sleeping 1 to 2 hours less per night than they need, according to a recent poll taken by the National Sleep Foundation. While insufficient sleep has often been associated with the elderly population, the increasing demands and lifestyles of modern society have imposed restricted sleep on our youth as well. . ."

COMMENT

This Editorial represents another important review of the dangers to health of short and poor quality sleep. The authors point out that American children are sleeping two hours less than required and that this alone is sufficient to promote a metabolic profile conducive to diabetes and obesity. The authors make no reference to the potential causes of this effect, and why poor quality/shortened sleep would impact the hormonal response, implicated in metabolic syndrome, but studies on raised cortisol and epinephrine (adrenal stress hormones) have been implicated in metabolic syndrome.

Replenishing the liver glycogen store prior to bedtime with honey may reduce the release of adrenal stress hormones overnight.

© Mike McInnes, MRPS and Ronald E Fessenden, MD, MPH, December 2007.

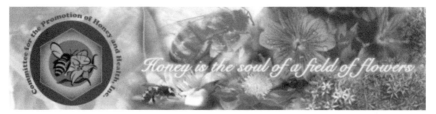

POSTER NO 6
Melatonin and Sleep - a Role for Honey

Pandi-Perumal SR, Srinivasan V, Maestroni GJ, Cardinali DP, Poeggeler B, Hardeland R, "Melatonin: Nature's most versatile biological signal?" **FEBS** Journal, Volume 273, Number 13, July 2006, pp. 2813-2838(26)

A Study from the Comprehensive Center for Sleep Medicine, Division of Pulmonary, Critical Care and Sleep Medicine, Mount Sinai School of Medicine, New York, NY 10029, USA.

SUMMARY

Melatonin is a ubiquitous molecule and widely distributed in nature, with functional activity occurring in unicellular organisms, plants, fungi and animals. In most vertebrates, including humans, melatonin is synthesized primarily in the pineal gland and is regulated by the environmental light/dark cycle via the suprachiasmatic nucleus. Pinealocytes function as 'neuroendocrine transducers' to secrete melatonin during the dark phase of the light/dark cycle and, consequently, melatonin is often called the 'hormone of darkness'. Melatonin is principally secreted at night and is centrally involved in sleep regulation, as well as in a number of other cyclical bodily activities. Melatonin is exclusively involved in signaling the 'time of day' and 'time of year' (hence considered to help both clock and calendar functions) to all tissues and is thus considered to be the body's chronological pacemaker or 'Zeitgeber'. Synthesis of melatonin also occurs in other areas of the body, including the retina, the gastrointestinal tract, skin, bone marrow and in lymphocytes, from which it may influence other physiological functions through paracrine signaling.

Melatonin has also been extracted from the seeds and leaves of a number of plants and its concentration in some of this material is several orders of magnitude higher than its night-time plasma value in humans. Melatonin participates in diverse physiological functions. In addition to its timekeeping functions, melatonin is an effective antioxidant which scavenges free radicals and up-regulates several antioxidant enzymes. It also has a strong antiapoptotic signaling function, an effect which it exerts even during ischemia. Melatonin's cytoprotective properties have practical implications in the treatment of neurodegenerative diseases. Melatonin also has immune-enhancing and oncostatic properties. Its 'chronobiotic' properties have been shown to have value in treating various circadian rhythm sleep disorders, such as jet lag or shift-work sleep disorder.

Melatonin acting as an 'internal sleep facilitator' promotes sleep, and melatonin's sleep-facilitating properties have been found to be useful for treating insomnia symptoms in elderly and depressive patients. A recently introduced melatonin analog, agomelatine, is also efficient for the treatment of major depressive disorder and bipolar affective disorder. Melatonin's role as a 'photoperiodic molecule' in seasonal reproduction has been established in photoperiodic species, although its regulatory influence in humans remains under investigation. Taken together, this evidence implicates melatonin in a broad range of effects with a significant regulatory influence over many of the body's physiological functions.

COMMENT

Melatonin is a multifaceted hormone that promotes sleep. Melatonin is also involved in immune function, anti-carcinogenic activity, anti-oxidant activity, anti-osteoporosis mechanisms, and may act as an anti-depressive hormone. The latest research on melatonin points to an important role in memory consolidation during rapid eye movement (REM) sleep.

Honey consumed prior to bedtime may promote sleep via release of melatonin as explained in the Honey - Insulin - Melatonin (HYMN) Cycle (see Poster No 14). Thus honey may be described as a natural facilitator or trigger for "optimized recovery physiology" during restorative sleep.

Appendix E

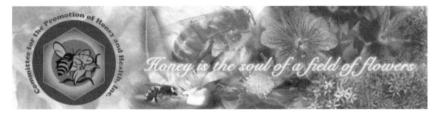

POSTER NO 7

Two Studies Relating Melatonin, Sleep and Memory Processes

Baydas G, Nedzvetsky VS, Nerush PA, Kirichenko SV, Demchenko HM, Reiter RJ. Neurosci Lett, "A novel role for melatonin: regulation of the expression of cell adhesion molecules in the rat hippocampus and cortex", **Neuroscience Letters**, 326(2):109-12, June 28, 2002.

Neural cell adhesion molecules (NCAMs) are members of the immunoglobulin superfamily and are involved in synaptic rearrangements in the mature brain. There are three major NCAM forms: NCAM 180, NCAM 140 and NCAM 120. Several studies report that NCAMs play a central role in memory. In the present study we investigated the effects of melatonin on the expression of NCAMs in the hippocampus, cortex and cerebellum. The levels of NCAMs were determined by Western blotting. After administration of melatonin for 7 days, NCAM 180 expression increased both in the hippocampus and in the cortex as compared to controls. On the contrary, in rats exposed to the constant light for 7 days (which inhibits endogenous production of melatonin), NCAM 180 levels decreased in the hippocampus and became undetectable in cortex and cerebellum. NCAM 140 levels were also diminished in the hippocampus of constant light-exposed rats. There was no change in NCAM 120 expression in any brain regions. This is the first report indicating that melatonin has a modulatory effect on the expression of NCAM in brain areas concerned with cognitive function. Melatonin may be involved in structural remodeling of synaptic connections during memory and learning processes.

Smith C, "Sleep states and memory processes", **Behavioral Brain Research**, 1995 Jul-Aug;69(1-2):137-45 from the Department of Psychology, Trent University, Peterborough, Ontario, Canada.

Evidence for the involvement of rapid eye movement (REM) sleep or paradoxical sleep (PS) with memory processing continues to accumulate. In animals, there is continuing evidence of relatively small, vulnerable paradoxical sleep windows (PSWs) following successful acquisition. These PSWs, which manifest as increases in PS over normal levels, appear to exhibit shorter latencies to onset when the amount of material presented during acquisition is increased. Prevention of the PSW results in memory deficits. In humans, there is now evidence that different types of tasks are differentially sensitive to rapid eye movement sleep deprivation REMD). Memory for declarative or explicit types of tasks, appears not to be affected by REM sleep loss, while memory for cognitive procedural or implicit types of material are impaired by REMD. Using post training auditory stimulation during REM sleep, memory enhancement of the procedural material is also possible. The memory for a fine motor task appears to be sensitive to post training stage 2 sleep loss. The important neural structures are generally not yet identifiable, although the hippocampus would appear to be important for place learning in the Morris water maze.

COMMENT

Rapid eye movement (REM) sleep is recognized as important for memory consolidation. Melatonin is emerging as critical for this vital physiology primarily for its modulatory effect on elaboration of neural cell adhesion molecules (NCAMs) during REM sleep. Melatonin appears to be involved in structural remodeling of synaptic connections during memory and learning processes via this mechanism.

Honey when consumed at bedtime will promote melatonin production via the HYMN cycle (see Poster No 14). Thus, honey may positively impact memory by two mechanisms: 1) by promoting melatonin which effects cognitive processes during REM sleep and 2) by reducing the production of the adrenal stress hormone, cortisol, which is known to attack short term memory in the hippocampus.

The Honey Revolution

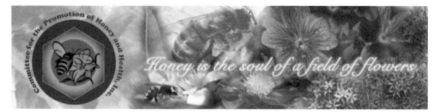

POSTER NO 8

Nighttime Caloric Intake is not Associated with Weight Gain

Sullivan, Elinor L; Daniels, Alejandro J; Koegler, Frank H; and Cameron, Judy L; "Evidence in Female Rhesus Monkeys (Macaca mulatta) that Nighttime Caloric Intake is not Associated with Weight Gain", **OBESITY RESEARCH**, Vol.13 No. 12:2072-2080 December 2005

ABSTRACT

Objective: To evaluate the hypothesis that nighttime consumption of calories leads to an increased propensity to gain weight.

Research Methods and Procedures: Sixteen female rhesus monkeys (Macaca mulatta) were ovariectomized and placed on a high-fat diet to promote weight gain, and we examined whether monkeys that ate a high percentage of calories at night were more likely to gain weight than monkeys that ate the majority of calories during the day.

Results: Within 6 weeks post-ovariectomy, calorie intake and body weight increased significantly (129 14%, p 0.04; 103 0.91%, p 0.02, respectively). Subsequent placement on high-fat diet led to further significant increases in calorie intake and body weight (368 56%, p 0.001; 113 4.0%, p 0.03, respectively). However, there was no correlation between the increase in calorie intake and weight gain (p 0.34). Considerable individual variation existed in the percentage of calories consumed at night (6% to 64% total daily caloric intake). However, the percentage of calorie intake occurring at night was not correlated with body weight (r 0.04; p 0.87) or weight gain (r 0.07; p 0.79) over the course of the study. Additionally, monkeys that showed the greatest nighttime calorie intake did not gain more weight (p 0.94) than monkeys that showed the least nighttime calorie intake.

Discussion: These results show that eating at night is not associated with an increased propensity to gain weight, suggesting that individuals trying to lose weight should not rely on decreasing evening calorie intake as a primary strategy for promoting weight loss.

Conclusion: In conclusion, our findings indicate that eating at night is not associated with increased propensity to gain weight. These results suggest that individuals trying to lose weight should not rely on decreasing evening calorie intake as a primary weight loss strategy but should focus on other strategies such as decreasing overall caloric intake and increasing activity level. . .

COMMENT

This elegant animal study demolishes the myth that "eating late turns to fat", a myth prevalent throughout western culture. Eating small portions before retiring has been known for many decades as part of the Mediterranean Diet. The benefits of this diet have been ignored in northern Europe and America. A large body of scientific literature focuses on the benefits of the Mediterranean Diet with respect to the types of food groups consumed. Little focus is given to the time of eating, the effect of liver glycogen replenishment prior to bedtime, and how this may positively impact both quality of sleep and recovery mechanisms during rest. This is strange because the relation between locomotion-food seeking (light) and sleep-satiety (dark) is well established in the literature as illustrated in this quote:

". . . Yet the evidence is increasingly strong that the neurophysiologic and metabolic mechanisms responsible for the control of food-seeking behavior and the control of sleep and wakefulness are coordinated so that hunger and vigilance are paired during the daylight hours, and satiety and sleep are paired during darkness."[1]

The key energy store during the night fast is the liver glycogen store, in so far as it must provide fuel for the brain over the 8 hour fast. Honey provides the perfect nutrient in terms of replenishing the liver glycogen store, and activating both sleep and recovery without digestive burden.

[1] Vantallie, Theodore B, From "Sleep and energy balance: interactive homeostatic systems", Metabolism Clinical and Experimental, 55 (supplement 2) (2006) s30-s35.

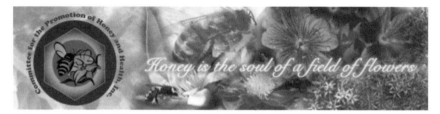

POSTER NO 9

The Significance of the Regulatory Effect of Liver Glycogen in Human Metabolism

Lavoie, Jean-Marc; Fillion, Yovan; Couturier, Karine; and Corriveau, Pierre; "Evidence that the decrease in liver glycogen is associated with the exercise-induced increase in IGFBP-1", **Journal of Applied Physiology** (May 3, 2002).

SUMMARY

The purpose of the present study was to test the hypothesis that exercise-induced increase in IGFBP-1 is not always linked to a decrease in blood glucose level and to examine if the decreasing levels of liver glycogen during exercise may be associated with the increase in IGFBP-1.

Three groups of rats were submitted to a 70-min treadmill exercise. One group of rats were (sic) normally fed and the two others had their food intake restricted by 50% (1/2 fast) the night before the experiment. One of these two 1/2 fasted groups of rats were infused (iv) with glucose throughout exercise to maintain euglycemia. Exercise in non-infused 1/2 fasted rats, compared to the normally fed rats, resulted in significant lower blood glucose (min 70) and insulin levels, and liver glycogen content, no change in IGF-I, and significant higher increases in FFA, glycerol, ß-hydroxybutyrate, and IGFBP-1. Maintenance of euglycemia during exercise in glucose-infused 1/2 fasted rats reduced to a large extent the decrease in insulin levels but only slightly attenuated the lipid response and the IGFBP-1 response seen in non-infused 1/2 fasted rats. Comparisons of all individual liver glycogen and IGFBP-1 values revealed that liver glycogen values were highly (P < 0.001) predictive of IGFBP-1 response during exercise (R = 0.564).

The present results indicate that IGFBP-1 response during exercise is not always linked to a decrease in plasma glucose and suggest that the increase in IGFBP-1 during exercise may be related to the decrease in liver glycogen content.

EDITOR'S COMMENT

Most of the work on liver glycogen was carried out in the first half of the twentieth century. Over the next five decades, this topic did not generate much scientific interest. This in itself is strange, in so far as liver glycogen is the primary reserve fuel store for the brain. The brain itself has no storage capacity for glucose (brain glucose will last only about 30 seconds under normal conditions). If and when liver glycogen runs low and is not adequately replenished, as during exercise and during the night fast, the brain activates the adrenal glands to release hormones which degrade tissue (mainly muscle protein) to create new glucose as fuel for liver replenishment. This animal study on liver glycogen depletion shows that even when blood glucose is stable, a signal is released from the liver (in the form of Insulin-like Growth Factor Binding Protein-1 or IGFBP-1) to "warn" the brain that trouble is ahead if action is not taken.

Another similar study indicates that IGFBP-1 is also released overnight.[1] In this study, the authors state that "insulin-like growth factor binding protein (IGFBP)-1 levels increase overnight, being inversely related to changes in insulin."

The Jean-Marc Lavoie study on exercise clearly shows the relation between liver glycogen plenitude and IGFBP-1 release. This relationship, along with the link in the second study to overnight physiology, indicates that this protein (IGFBP-1) is a stress signal from the liver indicating approaching metabolic danger to the brain, such as when the liver glycogen store is depleted. It is important to note again that the release of IGFBP-1 is independent of blood glucose levels. Liver depletion may occur when blood glucose is stable. In that case, if IGFBP-1 levels were linked only to blood glucose levels, liver depletion would *not* initiate a warning signal to the brain indicating an impending fuel shortage.

These studies underscore the need for selective replenishment of the liver prior to bedtime, especially when the evening meal is consumed much earlier. Honey is an ideal bedtime liver fuel as a tablespoon or two would provide the liver with sufficient fuel to stabilize blood glucose as well as maintain fuel supply to the brain during the eight hours of the night fast and thus reduce the production of the adrenal stress hormones, cortisol and adrenaline, that result over time, in chronic adrenal stress.

---

[1] Cotterill, AM; Holly, JM; Wass JA; "The regulation of insulin-like growth factor binding protein (IGFBP)-1 during prolonged fasting. Clinical Endocrinology (Oxford) 1993 Sep; 39(3): 357-62

© Mike McInnes, MRPS and Ronald E Fessenden, MD, MPH, December 2007.

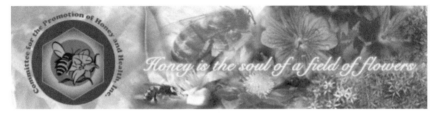

POSTER NO 10
Honey and Its Effect on the Immune System

Zidan, Jamal; Shetver, Lika; Gershuny, Anthony; Abzah, Amira; Tamam, Sigalit; Stein, Moshe; and Friedman, Eitan; "Prevention of Chemotherapy-Induced Neutropenia by Special Honey Intake", **American Journal of Clinical Nutrition**, Vol. 67, 519S-526S, Copyright © 1998 by The American Society for Clinical Nutrition, Inc. **Medical Oncology**, vol. 23, no. 4, 549-552, 2006

ABSTRACT

Febrile neutropenia is a serious side effect of chemotherapy. Colony-stimulating factors (CSFs) are used for primary and secondary treatment in patients with grade 4 neutropenia. The use of CSFs is expensive and accompanied by side effects. In the current study, Life-Mel Honey (LMH) was administered to prevent neutropenia and to reduce the need for CSFs in patients treated with chemotherapy. Thirty cancer patients receiving chemotherapy for primary or metastatic disease were included. All patients had grade 4 neutropenia and were treated with CSFs. The patients repeated the same chemotherapy schedule with the addition of LMH for 5 d. Blood count was performed weekly. There was no recurrence of neutropenia after LMH intake and no need for treatment with CSFs in 12 (40%) of patients. Eighteen (60%) patients with LMH developed neutropenia grade 4 and were treated with CSFs (p = 0.007). Hemoglobin levels remained >11 g/dL during LMH intake in 19 (64%) patients. Only three (10%) patients had thrombocytopenia. Eight (32%) patients reported improvement in quality of life. The use of LMH in patients who are at high risk of developing neutropenia as a result of chemotherapy decreases the risk of pancytopenia and the need for CSFs. LMH is inexpensive, has no side effects, and is easy to administer.

EDITOR'S COMMENT

This remarkable hospital-based study with human patients demonstrated that a special honey improved the immune system responses of patients undergoing chemotherapy for various types of cancer. In some study patients, the use of honey made the use of a drug (CSF) unnecessary (in the U.S., the cost of administration of CSF is over $1,000 per dose). That such a natural food may achieve such a powerful physiological effect is a significant demonstration of the potent and beneficial physiology of honey. The authors suggest that this effect is mediated by the antioxidant activity of honey. The antioxidant content of honey has been demonstrated in a number of studies and reports.

There may be other ways in which honey could affect immune function in such patients. Immunity is dependent on optimal cell metabolism, specifically muscle cells. Muscle cells supply the nutrients and energy necessary for rapid proliferation of immune cells during invasion or immune system compromise. If muscle cell metabolism is compromised, this will not happen optimally. We observe this in athletes who chronically over-train or fuel incorrectly. They suffer from compromised immune function, and are vulnerable to infections, particularly of the upper respiratory tract.

Other studies have also demonstrated that honey improves immune function.[1]

Honey taken prior to bed will boost the immune system by reducing production and release of cortisol, the stress hormone that attacks the immune system. Honey may also have a direct effect on elevating white cell counts and hemoglobin levels and decreasing IGE levels.[2]

[1] Al-Waili, Noori S, MD, "Effect of Honey on Antibody Production Against Thymus-Dependent and Thymus-Independent Antigens in Primary and Secondary Immune Responses", *Journal of Medicinal Foods*, 7 (4) 2004, 492–495

[2] Al-Waili, Noori S, MD, PhD, "Short Communication - Effects of Daily Consumption of Honey Solution on Hematological Indices and Blood Levels of Minerals and Enzymes in Normal Individuals", *Journal of Medicinal Foods*, Vol. 6, No 2, 2003

Appendix E

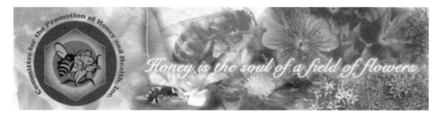

POSTER NO 11

Chronic Stress and Obesity: A New View of "Comfort Food"

Dallman, Mary F; Pecoraro, Norman; Akana, Susan F; la Fleur, Susanne E; Gomez, Francisca; Houshyar, Hani; Bell ME; Bhatnagar, Seema; Laugero, Kevin D; and Manalo, Sotara; "Chronic stress and obesity: A new view of 'comfort food'", Department of Physiology and Neuroscience Program, University of California, San Francisco, CA 94143-0444. [Communicated by Bruce S. McEwen, The Rockefeller University, New York, NY, July 28, 2003 (received for review May 14, 2003)]

ABSTRACT

The effects of adrenal corticosteroids on subsequent adrenocorticotropin secretion are complex. Acutely (within hours), glucocorticoids (GCs) directly inhibit further activity in the hypothalamo-pituitary-adrenal axis, but the chronic actions (across days) of these steroids on brain are directly excitatory. Chronically high concentrations of GCs act in three ways that are functionally congruent:

1. GCs increase the expression of corticotrophin-releasing factor (CRF) mRNA in the central nucleus of the amygdala, a critical node in the emotional brain. CRF enables recruitment of a chronic stress-response network.
2. GCs increase the salience of pleasurable or compulsive activities (ingesting sucrose, fat, and drugs, or wheel-running). This motivates ingestion of "comfort food."
3. GCs act systemically to increase abdominal fat depots. This allows an increased signal of abdominal energy stores to inhibit catecholamines in the brainstem and CRF expression in hypothalamic neurons regulating adrenocorticotropin.

Chronic stress, together with high GC concentrations, usually decreases body weight gain in rats; by contrast, in stressed or depressed humans chronic stress induces either increased comfort food intake and body weight gain or decreased intake and body weight loss. Comfort food ingestion that produces abdominal obesity, decreases CRF mRNA in the hypothalamus of rats. Depressed people who overeat have decreased cerebrospinal CRF, catecholamine concentrations, and hypothalamo-pituitary-adrenal activity. We propose that people eat comfort food in an attempt to reduce the activity in the chronic stress-response network with its attendant anxiety. These mechanisms, determined in rats, may explain some of the epidemic of obesity occurring in our society (emphasis added).

EDITOR'S COMMENT

The association of chronic adrenal stress with modern obesity is an important perspective to understand. Adrenal stress occurs in two primary situations: when liver glycogen stores are depleted due to prolonged exercise (or fasting) and near the end of the night fast when one goes to bed without replenishing liver glycogen stores. In addition, modern life styles frequently expose one to 24 hour day increased light pollution both within and without the home (cortisol is the only hormone directly stimulated by light). These conditions all militate against restful or restorative sleep.

Over time (months or years), this potent combination produces chronic adrenal stress and results in chronically distressed sleep, poor sleep architecture, compromised recovery and restoration of body tissues during rest, and inhibition of recovery fat metabolism, resulting in adult and childhood obesity.

Eating honey before bedtime insures adequate liver glycogen stores, improves sleep by virtue of the HYMN Cycle (see Poster NO 14), and improves sleep architecture. Individuals who consume a tablespoon or two of honey prior to bed often report increased dream memories. Dreams are a vital aspect of human sleep physiology and offline memory processing (see Poster NO 15). Honey before bedtime, it may be argued, is effective in promoting restorative sleep and reducing obesity by the mechanism of reducing or eliminating chronic adrenal stress.

The Honey Revolution

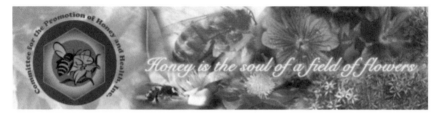

POSTER NO 12
Glucose vs. Fatty Acid Metabolism in the Human
- A model for Impaired Glucose Metabolism, Type II Diabetes, and Obesity

The following abstract advances a foundational shift in the rationale for the regulation of lipolysis and glycolysis in the human. Wolfe proposes that it is the availability of glucose or glycogen that controls fatty acid oxidation rather than the reverse hypothesis which had been held for over 35 years. When taken to the next logical step, Wolfe's mechanism or model better explains what happens with impaired glucose metabolism and the resultant development of type II diabetes and obesity. This understanding also underscores the role for honey in driving fat metabolism during rest and combating two key factors in the metabolic syndrome.

Wolfe, RR, "Metabolic interactions between glucose and fatty acids in humans", **American Journal of Clinical Nutrition**, Vol. 67, 519S-526S, © 1998 by The American Society for Clinical Nutrition, Inc.

ABSTRACT
In vivo energy production results largely from the oxidative metabolism of either glucose or fatty acids. Under diverse physiologic and nutritional conditions, the oxidation of either glucose or fatty acids may predominate. The nature of the control of the availability and oxidation of each substrate has been studied extensively for more than 30 years. The most popular and enduring hypothesis was proposed by Randle et al in 1963 and is termed the glucose-fatty acid cycle. This proposal places great significance on the regulation of lipolysis as a factor controlling substrate metabolism.

Key Steps:

Our work has led to an opposite perspective, which could be called the glucose-fatty acid cycle reversed. According to our hypothesis, the rate of glycolysis, determined by the intracellular availability of glucose-6-phosphate, is the predominant factor determining the rate of glucose oxidation. Whereas the rate of lipolysis may have some effect on the availability of glucose, both via a fatty acid-mediated inhibition of plasma glucose uptake and also by supplying glycerol for gluconeogenesis, there is little evidence for a direct inhibitory effect of fatty acid oxidation on the intracellular oxidation of glucose. In contrast, increased glucose oxidation limits oxidation of long-chain fatty acids directly by inhibiting their transport into the mitochondria.

Consequently, whereas there is a close coupling between glucose availability and oxidation, fatty acids are generally available in greater quantities than are required for oxidation. We propose that fatty acid oxidation is largely controlled at the site of oxidation, which is in turn determined by the availability of glucose, rather than by its availability via lipolysis.

EDITOR'S COMMENT
This review article, from 1998, is one of the seminal moments in 20th century metabolic science. Wolfe overturned one of the most important and widely held principles of metabolism of that century, the glucose-fatty acid cycle, which originated from Randle in 1963. This cycle was based on the notion that glucose metabolism is controlled by oxidation of fatty acids. Wolfe demonstrated that the opposite is the case and that metabolism of fatty acids is secondary to the metabolism of glucose.

If we factor in to this view the inhibition of glucose disposal by chronic stress which impairs glucose disposal, we have a model for type II diabetes and obesity. Chronic stress inhibits glucose metabolism and glucose disposal in cells. This in turn inhibits fat metabolism and disposal. The result is that both fuels, now considered excess energy intake by the human system, are stored as visceral fat (along with other consequences of the metabolic syndrome). By refueling liver glycogen and by improving glucose metabolism and disposal in peripheral cells, HONEY consumption (compared to other refined sugars) reduces metabolic stress and improves fat metabolism and disposal, thus combating two of the key parameters of metabolic syndrome, type II diabetes and obesity.

Model for Type II Diabetes and Obesity
Key Steps:
1. Glucose (glycogen) availability controls fatty acid oxidation (fat metabolism).
2. Chronic adrenal stress produces impaired glucose metabolism
3. Which in turn inhibits fat metabolism and disposal.
4. The result is the *Metabolic Syndrome* or Insulin Resistance with visceral obesity, increased risk of diabetes, CV disease and dyslipidemia.

Appendix E

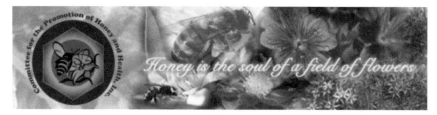

POSTER NO 13
The Importance of Adequate Liver Glycogen during Recovery Sleep

BULLOUGH, W S and EISA, E A, "The Diurnal Variations in the Tissue Glycogen Content and Their Relation to Mitotic Activity in the Adult Male Mouse", **Journal of Experimental Biology** 27,257-263 (1950), Published by Company of Biologists 1950, University of Sheffield, Farouk I University, Alexandria.

ABSTRACT

In a recent series of papers on the epidermis of the adult mouse (Bullough, 1949a, b, 1950a, b), it has been repeatedly stressed that the concentration of glucose or glycogen is the most important single factor affecting mitotic activity. In normal circumstances a high mitosis rate is seen only during rest or sleep, and it was suggested by Bullough (1949) that this may be related to the deposition of glucose from the blood at this time. While it is well known that most of the deposited glucose is stored in the liver in the form of glycogen, it also appeared possible that some may be stored on other tissues including the epidermis. Opportunity has now been found to check this hypothesis and to discover whether the diurnal rhythm in the glycogen content of the skin shows any relation to the diurnal rhythm in epidermal mitotic activity.

    1. A description is given of the hour-to-hour variation in the liver glycogen content in adult male mice, and it is shown that the concentration is highest while the animals are asleep and lowest while they are awake.

    2. A similar cycle is also described in the glycogen content of the skin. Histologically it is shown that a high proportion of the skin glycogen lies in the cytoplasm of the epidermal cells, and that during sleep both the epidermal glycogen content and the epidermal mitotic rate increase considerably. The skin glycogen content and the epidermal mitotic activity also show a marked increase after a subcutaneous injection of 20 mg. starch, while they are both abnormally depressed after two injections of 1/50 unit insulin.

    3. These results, together with others previously reported, are in agreement with the theory that at the onset of sleep glucose is deposited from the blood into the tissues where it appears in the form of glycogen. Since it is known that glucose, or glycogen, is a critical substance affecting mitotic activity in the adult mouse, it is logical to find that an increase in the epidermal glycogen content is accompanied by a greatly increased mitosis rate. On waking, the reverse process takes place, glycogen being withdrawn as glucose into the blood and mitotic activity falling to a low level.

EDITOR'S COMMENT

This dated but relevant study from 1950 shows that skin repair is cyclical and variant over time, correlated to sleep, and dependent on the glycogen content of the cell. The authors demonstrated that this content of cell glycogen is related directly to the content of liver glycogen. They show a clear correlation, at 2 hourly intervals over some 14 hours, between liver glycogen, tissue cell (in this case skin) glycogen, and mitosis (repair - formation of new cells).

We now know that when liver glycogen is low, repair of body cells (muscle, bone, and other body tissues) will be inhibited. The cascading steps are:

    1.   Low liver glycogen levels lead to
    2.   Release of cortisol which leads to
    3.   Release of IGFBP-1[1] (Insulin-like Growth Factor Finding Protein-1)

IGFBP-1 inhibits insulin-like growth factor-1, a key repair and recovery factor, which in humans is a sleep driven process. Thus, inadequate liver glycogen plenitude prior to bedtime will inhibit normal recovery and rebuilding of body cells/tissues. Consequently, less fat is burned during rest, since only "optimized recovery physiology" is fat fueled physiology.

Liver glycogen may be selectively replenished prior to bed with honey, inhibiting IGFBP-1 release. The result will be improved sleep, improved recovery/rebuilding of body tissues, reduction of adrenal stress overnight, and optimal fat metabolism (increased fat-burning).

Honey is the perfect food for liver replenishment prior to bed and for activating sleep and optimizing recovery physiology.

[1]Conover et al, "Cortisol increases plasma insulin-like growth factor binding protein-1 in humans", **Acta Endocrinol** (Copenhagen). 1993 Feb;128 (2):140-3).

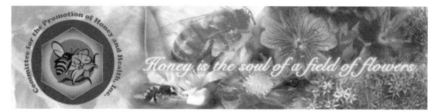

POSTER NO 14

HONEY, SLEEP AND THE "HYMN" CYCLE

Honey may improve sleep quality. The mechanism for this can be described in what the editors call the **Honey-Insulin-Melatonin Cycle** or "HYMN" Cycle.

Each individual step of the cycle is well established and may be found in routine text books of biochemistry. Together, these steps describe a cycle of metabolic activity that culminates in "optimized recovery physiology" during "restorative sleep", and more importantly in the reduction in the release of stress hormones during the night fast. **The cycle begins with the ingestion of 1 to 2 tablespoons of honey in the hour prior to bedtime and proceeds as follows:**

1. The glucose moiety (portion) of honey passes from the gut, through the liver circulation and into the general circulation producing a mild glucose spike. (Glucose from honey produces only a mild or controlled elevation in blood sugar primarily because the fructose moiety facilitates glucose uptake into the liver where it is converted to glycogen. Thus less glucose reaches or remains in the general circulation.)
2. **The mild elevation in blood sugar (from glucose) prompts a mild controlled release of insulin from the pancreas.**
3. The presence of insulin in the general circulation drives tryptophan into the brain.
4. **Tryptophan is converted to serotonin, a key hormone that promotes relaxation.**
5. In darkness, serotonin is converted to melatonin in the pineal gland.
6. **Melatonin activates sleep (by reducing body temperature and other mechanisms).**
7. Melatonin also inhibits the release of more insulin from the pancreas – an example of the wonderfully creative "feedback" or control mechanism of the Hymn Cycle – thus preventing a rapid drop in blood sugar level.
8. **Melatonin promotes the release of growth hormone by another of the curious and round-about routes that the human system excels in. The release of growth hormone is controlled by the activity of a growth-hormone-releasing hormone. This hormone is turn inhibited by another hormone - growth-hormone-releasing-hormone inhibiting hormone. Melatonin inhibits this last hormone, thus preventing the inhibition of growth hormone releasing hormone, and therefore promoting the release of growth hormone from the pituitary gland. Growth hormone is the hormone governing all of recovery physiology. This is the key first step in recovery or restorative physiology that occurs overnight.**
9. Next, a cascade of recovery hormones initiate the repair, maintenance and rebuilding of bone, muscle, and other body tissues. NOTE: For "optimized recovery" to take place, there must be sufficient glycogen stores in the liver. When liver glycogen stores are adequate, "optimized recovery physiology" is almost exclusively fat-burning physiology. Although this seems counterintuitive, the science that documents the burning of fat during rest is well established.
10. **Melatonin also impacts memory consolidation by its requirement for the formation of NCAMS - neural cell adhesion molecules - during REM sleep - and these are necessary for the processing of short term memory from the hippocampus into long term memory in the brain cortex.**
11. Concurrent with the above, the fructose moiety of honey carries out its critical role. Fructose is taken up by the liver where some is converted to glucose and then to liver glycogen, thus providing the brain with a sustained supply of glucose for the night fast. (Without liver glycogen for fuel, the brain only has sufficient glycogen to survive about 30 seconds.)
12. **Additionally, fructose regulates glucose uptake into the liver by prompting release of glucokinase from the hepatocyte nuclei. Glucokinase is found primarily in the liver cell nuclei and is necessary for the conversion of glucose to glycogen. This action of fructose in releasing glucokinase is a wondrous metabolic phenomenon we term "The Fructose Paradox". Thus, fructose insures good liver glycogen supply overnight and prevents a major glucose/insulin spike as referred to in #1 above.**
13. An adequate liver glycogen supply means that stress hormones (released to maintain fuel supply to the brain in the absence of adequate liver glycogen) need not be released. This exceedingly beneficial effect on an individual's hormone profile over time will have a profound impact on the public health concerns regarding obesity, diabetes and other metabolic conditions. **NOTE: In northern Europe and America, the notion that we should not eat before bedtime results in chronic release of adrenal hormones during rest, impacting sleep architecture and resulting over time, in increased risk of heart disease, hypertension, osteoporosis, diabetes, obesity, gastric ulcers, childhood obesity, depression, memory loss and dementias - all conditions associated with chronic release of adrenal hormones.**

Application and Conclusion: After an early evening meal, a tablespoon or two of honey prior to bed will activate the sleep cycle and the recovery cycle. With the consumption of honey before bedtime, sleep quality is improved, recovery (fat burning) physiology is optimized, and the chronic release of adrenal stress hormones is inhibited. It is postulated that by the mechanisms articulated above, the effect will be a reduction in the risk for all the diseases associated with metabolic syndrome referred to in 13 above.

Additional References:
1) Murray RK, Granner DK, Mayes PA, Rodwell, VW, **Harper's Biochemistry,** 22nd Edition, Appleton & Lange,1990
2) Rang HP, Dale MM, **Pharmacology,** Churchill Livingstone, Edinburgh, 1991.
3) Gibney MJ, Macdonald IA, Roche HM, **Nutrition & Metabolism,** Blackwell Publishing, Oxford 2003.

Appendix E

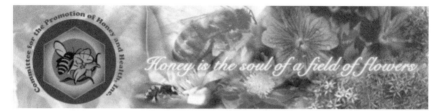

POSTER NO 15

The following are selected portions of published Abstracts relating to Sleep Physiology, Off-line Memory Processing and Dream Psychology. The research presented in these articles frames the argument and underscores the rationale for "fueling" the liver at bedtime to insure an adequate glycogen supply for the overnight fast. Honey is proposed as the ideal bedtime liver fuel.

Physiology of Sleep and Psychology of Dreams

AS, Eiser, **Seminal Neurology**, March; 25(1): 97-105

"The discovery of the close association between rapid eye movement (REM) sleep and dreaming and the development of sleep laboratory techniques ushered in a new era in the study of dreams . . . Some **more recent theories of dreaming emphasize an adaptive function related to emotion and a role in learning and memory consolidation** (emphasis added)."

Sleep, Dreams, and Memory Consolidation

Payne, Jessica D, and Nadel, Lynn, "Sleep, dreams, and memory consolidation: the role of the stress hormone cortisol", **LEARNING & MEMORY** 11:671-678; © 2004 by Cold Spring Harbor Laboratory Press; ISSN 1072-0502/04

"In addition to clinical evidence, there is experimental evidence that high levels of cortisol alter memory function. Patient populations with chronically elevated levels of cortisol, such as Cushing's syndrome, major depression, and schizophrenia, as well as asthmatic patients treated with the glucocorticoid prednisone are characterized by impaired memory function . . . not surprisingly, however, REM sleep in patients with Cushing's syndrome is strikingly similar to the sleep of patients with major depression, with REM latency being shortened and REM density being increased (see Shipley et al. 1992)."

Schizophrenia – a Diabetic Brain State

Holden, R J and Mooney, P A, "Schizophrenia is a diabetic brain state: an elucidation of impaired neuro-metabolism", **Med-Hypotheses**, 1994 Dec; 43(6): 420-35

"In this paper a detailed argument will be advanced in support of the notion that schizophrenia is fundamentally a diabetic brain state, henceforth referred to as 'cerebral diabetes'. In so doing, we shall provide a metabolic explanation for all the prominent symptoms currently known to be associated with cerebral diabetes and indicate some future therapeutic interventions."

Sleep - - Off-line Memory Processing

Stickgold R, Hobson JA, Fosse R, Fosse M, "Sleep, learning, and dreams: off-line memory reprocessing", **Science**, 2001 Nov 2; 294(5544):1052-7

"Converging evidence and new research methodologies from across the neurosciences permit the neuroscientific study of the role of sleep in off-line memory reprocessing, as well as the nature and function of dreaming. Evidence supports a role for sleep in the consolidation of an array of learning and memory tasks (emphasis added). In addition, new methodologies allow the experimental manipulation of dream content at sleep onset, permitting an objective and scientific study of this dream formation and a renewed search for the possible functions of dreaming and the biological processes sub-serving it."

EDITOR'S COMMENT

One of the most consistent anecdotal reports received from those who take a dose of honey prior to bed, is that of improved quality of sleep and increased dream recall. It's "like watching cable TV" one person commented. It is becoming clearer that dreams are not only essential for memory processing, they are critical to human psychological and physical health.

Impaired memory processing has been related to Cushing's syndrome, depression and schizophrenia. That schizophrenia has been characterized as a "diabetic brain state" and related to chronically elevated levels of cortisol, as in classical type 2 diabetes and insulin resistance in muscle, is consistent with the model of modern obesity and diabetes. These latter conditions are characterized by chronic cortisol-induced impairment of glucose metabolism and disposal, leading to impaired fat metabolism. When fat metabolism is impaired, both fuels - glucose and fats - are stored as abdominal fat manifesting a kind of reverse metabolism.

The editors postulate that honey may be shown to drive metabolism forward, resulting in increased fat metabolism during rest by virtue of improved hepatic and muscle cell metabolism assisted by the glucins. Overnight, in particular, honey may be the ideal fuel for improved quality of sleep, facilitating "off-line memory processing", and enhancing REM sleep and dream induction. By reducing or eliminating chronic overproduction of cortisol, honey may be found to contribute to an improved psychology of dreams along with improved physiology of sleep.

© Mike McInnes, MRPS and Ronald E Fessenden, MD, MPH, December 2007.

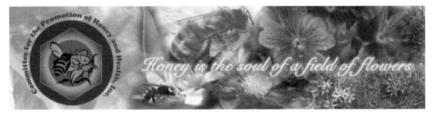

POSTER NO 16
Honey, Mental Fatigue (Neurasthenia) and Physical Fatigue (Myasthenia)

Professor Anson Rabinach, in *The Human Motor* [1], describes how, in the late 19th century, there developed a wide academic movement interested in physical fatigue and what was then described as neurasthenia (mental fatigue). Physicians, physiologists, researchers and scholars, from a variety of scientific disciplines, studied physical and mental fatigue, from differing perspectives. There was much concern from teachers, employers, government and magistrates, about the increasing intellectual burden imposed on the new generations of students, resulting from the leap forward in all the sciences, and the vast accumulation in knowledge, required by students to keep pace with rapid developments in science and technology. It was considered that this explosion of knowledge would overwhelm students, and that this may threaten the ability of the state to find politicians, bureaucrats, officials, technicians, teachers, lecturers, lawyers and other professional workers, who would be able to absorb, master and use this exponentially increasing body of knowledge, to maintain and administer the growing urban and advanced society, without suffering breakdown from mental exhaustion (neurasthenia).

In modern times we may call this stress, but the mental and physical physiology studied by these pioneers, is the broadly similar. The overall theory is not radically different from our approach today and learning/memory consolidation and retrieval are known to be intimately correlated with, and modulated by, stress physiology.

In Oxford in the1640's, an English physician, Thomas Willis[2] wrote about what he termed the *incorporeal* aspect of humans, as opposed to the *corporeal*. By *incorporeal* he referred to the mind, as opposed to the body. Not only did he separate the two, he described them as in *conflict*. Modern physiology agrees with this. **During exercise, contracting muscles extract glucose from the circulation, and this glucose, which is released from the liver, is actually fuel required by the brain. It is therefore perfectly correct to state that during exercise, brain and muscles compete for the same fuel source, liver glycogen (glucose), and as muscles increase this extraction, the brain is placed at risk.** As the liver store depletes and glucose is increasingly used by contracting muscles, there is a very real danger of blood glucose falling to below normal levels. This indeed does occur when athletes collapse.

APPLICATION AND CONCLUSION

There is a common link in the "liver-brain axis" to both exercise and sleep. During exercise, contracting muscles extract glucose from the circulation and blood sugar levels fall. During a typical 8 hour night fast, blood sugar levels may drop below normal if the small liver glycogen store is not restocked just prior to bedtime. *Both situations result in excess production and release of adrenal stress hormones, with negative impacts on health.*

It seems that both athletes/coaches and the general population appear to be 'liver blind' with respect to the importance of maintaining an adequate liver glycogen store. Athletes must fuel their liver before, during and after exercise, and prior to overnight recovery or *pay a heavy price in terms of performance, recovery and general health.* The general population must resist the notion of "not eating before bedtime" which risks having a depleted liver and *results in poor recovery, poor sleep quality, and a negative metabolic profile which when repeated over several years may contribute to hypertension, cardiovascular disease, obesity and diabetes.*
Honey, with its powerful metabolic profile and potential, is an excellent fuel for both exercise and restorative sleep. Honey, because of its rapid incorporation into liver glycogen, provides a simple, natural solution for neurasthenia and myasthenia, a fatigued mind and body.

[1] Rabinach, Anson, **The Human Motor,** University of California Press 1992, © 1990 by Basic Books Inc.
[2] Willis, Thomas, **Bodies/Minds,** Edited by Iwan Rhys Morus in 'A Great and Difficult Thing': Understanding and Explaining the Human Machine in Restoration England', Chapter 2; Michael Hawkins, 2002, Berg Oxford

Appendix F - Glossary

Adrenal Glands: The adrenal glands are two hat-shaped glands that sit above each kidney. Upon receiving signals from the brain during stress they release two key hormones, adrenaline and cortisol. These hormones are typically described as fight/flight hormones in the literature, but this is technically incorrect. Rather these hormones should be viewed as neuroprotective hormones in so far as they retain glucose in the circulation by inhibiting muscle uptake of glucose. Thus the fuel supply to the brain is maintained during times when the brain is at risk.

Adrenaline: Adrenaline (or epinephrine as it is known in the U.S.) is a stress hormone released by the adrenal glands during so-called fight/flight episodes. It is a sympathomimetic hormone (or catecholamine). Adrenaline raises blood glucose concentration, increases blood pressure and heart rate, thereby increasing the supply of glucose and oxygen to the brain. Like cortisol it is essentially a neuroprotective hormone, and is released during episodes when brain metablolosm is at risk. Another sympathomimetic hormone known as noradrenaline is released in the brain, and mimics adrenaline in its actions in the body. In The Honey Revolution these two similar hormones are not distinguished but readers should be aware that there are some differences in action.

11BetaHSD-1: The enzyme (11Beta Hydroxysteroid Dehydrogenase-1) converts inactive cortisone to active cortisol within the cells. The enzyme is controlled by IFG-1, which lowers the activity of 11BetaHSD-1 reducing intracellular metabolic stress. 11BetaHSD-1 is emerging as an important player in diabetes and other conditions of the metabolic syndrome and pharmaceutical companies and other researchers are investigating drugs whose function is to antagonise this enzyme.

Cortisol: Cortisol is a steroid stress hormone, released from the adrenal glands during so-called fight/flight episodes. It is a glucoregulatory hormone and raises blood glucose concentration by promoting conversion of degraded muscle protein to glucose in the liver (gluconeogenesis) which in turn promotes the formation of liver glycogen. Although it is usually referred to as a fight/flight hormone, it is more correctly termed a neuroprotective hormone. Chronic overproduction of cortisol results in conditions associated with metabolic syndrome.

Fructokinase: Fructokinase is an enzyme in the cytosol of liver cells (hepatocytes).   Fructokinase allows for optimal uptake of fructose into the liver and regulates glucose uptake, by allowing for fructose driven liberation of glucokinase (the Fructose Paradox). This mechanism insures and reserves fuel supply for the brain when it is at risk.

Fructose: Fructose is a six carbon monnosaccharide that is central to human energy metabolism.   This sugar is taken up by liver cells, by virtue of the enzyme fructokinase, and is converted to glucose and liver glycogen. Fructose regulates glucose uptake and metabolism in liver cells, and this function is vital for reserving fuel supply for the brain when this is at risk. Fructose in nature is found in fruits, vegetables and honey, almost always in a near 1:1 ratio with glucose and/or other sugars.

Glucagon: Glucagon is a hormone produced and released by the pancreas when blood glucose concentration is low.   Its acts mainly in the liver where it causes the breakdown of liver glycogen so that glucose may be released into the circulation.   It acts in opposition to insulin.   Glucagon is the hormone associated with morning sickness, and may be viewd as a stress hormone associated with metabolic stress, when brain metablism is at risk.

Glycogen: Glycogen is stored glucose in cells, particularly in muscle and liver.   This form of storage packs long chain glucose molecules into small volume storage, similar to starch in plant cells.   Muscle glycogen is selectively reserved to provide glucose for contracting muscles cells where it is metabolized during exercise.   Liver glycogen is stored and released into the circulation when blood glucose levels fall.   Its primary role is to provide a reserve fuel supply for the brain especially during periods when the brain is placed at risk, such as during exercise and during the night fast.

Insulin: Insulin is a hormone produced and released from the pancreas gland that regulates blood glucose.   When glucose levels rise in the circulation insulin stimulates muscle, liver and fat cells to take in glucose.   Muscle and liver cells utilise the glucose or store it as glycogen (starch).   Fat cells use glucose as a storage molecule for fats by splitting glucose to form glycerol. Insulin is responsible both for the storage of fat and for promoting the formation of amino acids into proteins. Thus it is known both as a storage and building hormone.

Glucokinase: Glucokinase is the enzyme required for glucose uptake into the liver cells. However, in the post meal period, glucokinase remains locked in the liver cell nucleus (unlike fructokinase) and is not available to assist in glucose uptake.   Small concentrations of fructose liberate glucokinase from the liver cell nuclei and allow for glucose uptake into liver.

Hepathlete: A hepathlete is a liver conscious athlete.

Hypothalamus: The hypothalamus links the brain (the central nervous system) to the body via the pituitary gland and the endocrine system. It is located just above the brain stem and releases hormones which control the pituitary gland which is the master endocrine gland. The hypothalamus is intimately involved in energy homeostasis, and controls all our most fundamental physiological drives such as hunger, thirst, energy partition and use, circadian cycles, emotions and temperature regulation.

IGF-1: IGF-1 or Insulin Like Growth factor-1, is an important growth hormone during childhood and during periods of recovery in adults. It also acts as a powerful insulin signalling hormone.

IGFBP-1: IGFBP-1 or Insulin Like Growth Factor Binding Protein-1 is a protein released from the liver when liver glycogen is low. IGFBP-1 acts both as a signal to the brain and as a stress hormone that acts to inhibit glucose disposal into tissues. It does this by binding and inhibiting IGF-1, an insulin signalling hormone. Thus IGFBP-1 functions as an important glucoregulatory principle.

Liver: The liver is one of the most important internal organs in the human body. It is involved in appetite control, food and energy processing and partition, protein and fat synthesis, detoxification, bile formation and deconstruction of red blood cells. It plays a critical role in maintaining fuel supply to the brain from its small glycogen store either by releasing stored glucose from glycogen (glycogenolysis) or by constructing new glucose from degraded muscle protein (gluconcogenesis). It is the only organ in the body with the enzyme required to release glucose into the circulation. This role becomes vital during times when glucose supply to the brain may be compromised, such as during exercise and during the night fast.

Liver Blindness: Liver blindness is a scientific/cultural form of blindness, that results from the lack of interest in liver glycogen in medical and sport science faculties. This critically important fuel store plays an important role during exercise and recovery. To that extent that the liver may be regarded as the key organ of exercise and recovery.

Maltodextrins: Maltodextrins are long chain glucose polymers produced from starch. They are hydrolysed in the human intestine to free glucose, which is then absorbed into the circulation. They are widely used in sport to provide fuel for contracting muscles, before and during exercise. It is important for athletes to keep in mind that without the presence of fructose in the fuel, little or no glucose uptake into liver will take place, and metabolic stress will be initiated. Glucose and/or glucose polymers will fuel contracting muscles, but this ignores the critical role of fructose in the liver/brain axis.

Metabolic Stress: Metabolic stress is the result of activation of a cascade of stress hormones from the hypothalamus and the pituitary gland (the HPA axis) and involving release of adrenal stress hormones. This cascade is most often referred to in periods of hypoglycemia (low blood glucose) but is now increasingly correlated with low liver glycogen status, and release of the stress protein IGFBP-1.

Metabolic Syndrome: the metabolic syndrome, also known as Syndrome X, is a series of conditions associated with chronic overproduction of adrenal stress hormones. The best known of these conditions are cardiovascular disease and diabetes, but the syndromes are now being expanded to include obesity, gastric ulcers, osteoporosis, infertility, memory loss, depression, dementias and Alzheimer's disease. The metabolic syndrome is thought to affect 25% of the American population.

Pineal Gland: The pineal gland is a pine cone shaped endocrine gland in the rear of the brain. This vital gland releases melatonin, an important hormone that regulates sleep in humans. Melatonin is profoundly involved in memory processing and is required for processing short term into long term memory during REM sleep.

Pituitary Gland: The pituitary gland is a small endocrine gland that is connected to the hypothalamus, near the base of the brain. The hypothalamus controls the pituitary gland by releasing a series of controlling hormones, both stimulating and inhibitory. The pituitray is divided into two regions, the anterior and the posterior. The key hormones of the anterior pituitary are ACTH (adrenocorticotrophic hormone) which controls the adrenal glands, and growth hormones which controls growth and recovery. Other hormones are TSH (thyroid stimulating hormone), prolactin, endorphins, FSH (follicle stimulating hormone) and LH (leutenizing hormone). The posterior pituitary releases oxytocin, and vasopressin. The significant hormones with respect to The Honey Revolution are ACTH and growth hormone.

Slow Wave Sleep: Slow wave sleep (or non-rapid eye movement sleep) refers to the periods of deepest sleep and is associated with optimum recovery physiology. It comprises two stages, and ocurrs mainly in the first four hours of sleep. The second four hours of sleep are characterised by increased arousal, and are the period when the body is preparing for the following day. In this period circadian cycling is associated with release of adrenal hormones, in particular cortisol, which is also stimulated by early morning light.

Stress: Stress results from inability of an organism to adapt to rapid alterations in the environment.   Rapid changes in the flux of fuels, nutrients and oxygen and thermoregulation place acute demand on homeostasis, and stress is the attempt to regain homeostic competence.   Stress may result from psychological, physiologial (metabolic), physical or environmental stimuli.

Suprachiasmatic Nucleus (SCN):   The SCN is located in the hypothalamus, functions as the central body clock, and regulates circadian rythms.   It is important for regulation of fuel homeostasis, partitioning between locomotion/ food seeking and sleep/energy status.

The Fructose Paradox: The Fructose Paradox refers to the liberation of glucokinase from the liver cell nucleus by fructose.   When fructose is taken into liver cells, by virtue of fruktokinase, it liberates the glucose enzyme, glucokinase and this in turn allows for liver uptake of glucose.   This exquisite regulation of glucose metabolism by fructose is one of the most important and least appreciated mechanisms of central energy metabolism in humans, and if optimal sequesters fuel supply for the brain.

The Glucose Paradox: The Glucose Paradox, first postulated by Katz and McGarry in an iconic paper (The Glucose Paradox 1986), describes the notion that glucose is not a good substrate for uptake into liver cells or for the formation of liver glycogen.   The idea was first hinted at by Claude Bernard, who discovered liver glycogen, in the 19th century.

End Notes

Introduction

[1] Medical obesity may be determined by calculating one's Body Mass Index (BMI). BMI is defined as individual's body weight divided by the square of their height as stated in kg/m^2 A number above 30 suggests that a person is obese. A number above 40 indicates morbid obesity.

[2] The *metabolic syndrome* is a combination of medical disorders that increase the risk of developing cardiovascular disease and diabetes. It affects a large number of people, and prevalence increases with age. Some studies estimate the prevalence in the USA to be up to 25% of the population. Symptoms and features of metabolic syndrome include:

- Insulin resistance, fasting hyperglycemia, diabetes mellitus type 2 or impaired fasting glucose, impaired glucose tolerance;
- Hypertension or elevated blood pressure;
- Central obesity (also known as visceral, male-pattern or apple-shaped adiposity), overweight with fat deposits mainly around the waist;
- Decreased HDL cholesterol;
- Elevated triglycerides;
- And other associated diseases and signs including elevated uric acid levels, fatty liver (especially in concurrent obesity), progressing to non-alcoholic fatty liver disease, polycystic ovarian syndrome, hemochromatosis (iron overload), and acanthosis nigricans (a skin condition featuring dark patches).

[Taken from: Alberti KG, Zimmet P, Shaw J, "Metabolic syndrome-a new world-wide definition, A Consensus Statement from the International Diabetes Federation," **Diabetic Medicine** 2006 May; 23(5): 469-80.]

[3] Basciano H, Federico L, Adeli K, "Fructose, insulin resistance, and metabolic dyslipidemia." **Nutr Metab** (London) 2005 Feb 21; 2(1): 5

[4] Ravi Dhingra, MD, *et.al.*, "Soft Drink Consumption and Risk of Developing Cardiometabolic Risk Factors and the Metabolic Syndrome in Middle-Aged Adults in the Community," **Circulation** 2007; 116: 480-488

[5] George A Bray, Samara Joy Nielsen, and Barry M Popkin, "Consumption of high-fructose corn syrup in beverages may play a role in the epidemic of obesity," **Am J Clin Nutr** 2004;79:537– 43. Printed in USA. © 2004 American Society for Clinical Nutrition

Chapter 1

[6] Nectar contains varying amounts of glucose, fructose and sucrose depending on the floral source. Honeybees prefer mixtures of different sugars rather than nectars in which only one of the sugars predominates, choosing richer nectars which have more than 15% sugar.

[7] The actual ratio of fructose to glucose varies among honey varietals from .98 to 1.5 depending on the sucrose content of the nectar on which the honeybee forages.

[8] Dick Paetzke, 1987

Chapter 2

[9] Randle PJ, Garland PB, Hales CN, Newsholme EA, "The glucose fatty-acid cycle. Its role in insulin sensitivity and the metabolic disturbances of diabetes mellitus." (1963) **Lancet 1**: 785-9

[10] Wolfe, RR, "Metabolic interactions between glucose and fatty acids in humans." **American Journal of Clinical Nutrition**, Vol. 67, 519S-526S Copyright © 1998 by The American Society for Clinical Nutrition, Inc

[11] Rizza, RA, Mandarino, LJ and Gerich, J, "Cortisol-induced insulin resistance in man: impaired suppression of glucose production and stimulation of glucose utilization due to a postreceptor defect of insulin action." **J Clin Endocrinol Metab** (1982) 54, 131-138

[12] Bjorntorp, P., "Visceral fat accumulation: the missing link between psychosocial factors and cardiovascular disease?" **J Intern Med** (1991) 230, 195-201

[13] Dallman, M.F., Strack, A.M., Akana, S.F. et al, "Feast and famine: critical role of glucocorticoids with insulin in daily energy flow." **Front Neuroendocrinol** (1993) 14, 303-347

[14] Dinneen, S., Alzaid, A., Miles, J. and Rizza, R., "Metabolic effects of the nocturnal rise in cortisol on carbohydrate metabolism in normal humans." **J Clin Invest** (1993) 92, 2283-2290

[15] Andrews R.C, Walker B.R., "Glucocorticoids and insulin resistance: old hormones, new targets." **Clinical Science** (1999) 96, pp. 513-523

[16] Ibid, Wolfe, RR

[17] Food and Nutrition Board (2002/2005). Dietary Reference Intakes for Energy, Carbohydrate, Fiber, Fat, Fatty Acids, Cholesterol, Protein, and Amino Acids. Washington, DC: The National Academies Press. Page 769

[18] Joint WHO/FAO expert consultation (2003). Diet, Nutrition and the Prevention of Chronic Diseases (PDF). Geneva: World Health Organization. pp. 55-56

[19] Robert C Atkins, MD with Sheila Buff, "Dr. Atkins' Age-Defying Diet Revolution," 2000 St. Martin's Press, p. 8 cited from Castelli, WP, "Concerning the possibility of a nutritional . . ." **Arch Intern Med** 1992; 152: 1371-72

[20] The fact that ingestion of saturated fats cannot be associated with elevated cholesterol levels (though there continues to be debate on the subject of saturated fats and cholesterol profiles) should not infer that saturated fats are not associated with coronary heart disease and atherosclerosis. The challenge for much of the world's scientific research and literature in this matter is controlling for sugar intake. Excessive sugar ingestion over time impairs glucose metabolism which in turn inhibits fat metabolism and fat disposal.

[21] Del Prete E, Lutz TA, Althaus J, and Scharrer E, "Inhibitors of fatty acid oxidation (mercaptoacetate, R-3-amino-4- trimethylaminobutyric acid) stimulate feeding in mice." (1998) **Physiol Behav** 63: 751–754

[22] Lands, William EM, "Biosynthesis of Prostaglandins." **Ann Rev Nutr** (1991) University of Chicago, pp. 1141-60

[23] Ibid, Wolfe, RR.

[24] Wolfe, RR, Klein, S, Carraro, F, Weber, J M, "Role of triglyceride-fatty acid cycle in controlling fat metabolism in humans during and after exercise," **Am J Physiol** 1990, 258, E382-E389

[25] JF Brun, M Dumortier, C Fedou, J Mercier, "Exercise hypoglycaemia in non diabetic subjects." **Diabetes Metab** (Paris) 2001, 27, 92-106

[26] "Fat to the fire: The regulation of lipid oxidation with exercise and environmental stress." Grant B Mc Lelland Company, **Biochem and Physiol** Part B 139: pp. 443-460

[27] Atkins, Robert C, MD, "**Dr. Atkins' New Diet Revolution**," St, Martin's Press, New York

[28] Jenni L, Jenni-Eirman S, Spina F, Schwabl H, "Regulation of protein breakdown and adrenocortical responses to stress in birds during migratory flight." **Am J Physiol Regul Integr Comp Physiol** 2000 May; 278(5): RI1182-9

[29] Each gram of glucose provides 4 Calories of energy requirement.

[30] Mark Hyman, MD, **Ultrametabolism**, Scribner, 2006 and **The Ultrametabolism Cookbook**, Scribner, 2007

Chapter 3

[31] L.M. CHEPULIS, "The Effect of Honey Compared to Sucrose, Mixed Sugars, and a Sugar-Free Diet on Weight Gain in Young Rats," **Journal of Food Science**, 1750-3841, 2007

[32] G.B.K.S. Prasad, et al, "Subjects with Impaired Glucose Tolerance Exhibit a High Degree of Tolerance to Honey," **J Med Food** 10 (3) 2007, 473–478

[33] Samanta A, Burden AC, Jones GR, "Plasma glucose responses to glucose, sucrose, and honey in patients with diabetes mellitus: an analysis of glycaemic and peak incremental indices." **Diabet Med**, 1985 Sep; 2(5): 371-3

[34] Ibid

[35] Ibid, G.B.K.S. Prasad, et al

[36] Guidi I, Galimberti D, Lonati S, Novembrino C, Bamonti F, Tiriticco M, Fenoglio C, Venturelli E, Baron P, Bresolin N, Scarpini E., "Oxidative imbalance in patients with mild cognitive impairment and Alzheimer's disease," **Neurobiol Aging** 2006 Feb; 27(2): 262-9

[37] Messier C., "Impact of impaired glucose tolerance and Type 2 Diabetes on cognitive aging." **Neurobiol Aging** 2005 Dec; 26 Suppl 1: 26-30

[38] Awad N, Gagnon M, Messier C., "The relationship between impaired glucose tolerance, Type 2 Diabetes, and cognitive function." **J Clin Exp Neuropsychol** 2004 Nov; 26(8): 1044-80

[39] Pasquier F, Boulogne A, Leys D, Fontaine P, "Diabetes mellitus and dementia." **Diabetes Metab** 2006 Nov; 32 (5 Pt 1): 403-14

[40] Ibid, Awad and Messier

[41] Messier C, Awad N, Gagnon M., "The relationships between atherosclerosis, heart disease, Type 2 Diabetes and dementia," **Neurol Res** 2004 Jul; 26(5): 567-72

[42] Busserolles, Jérôme; Gueux, Elyett; Rock, Edmond; Mazur, Andrzej and Rayssiguier, Yves; "Substituting Honey for Refined Carbohydrates Protects Rats from Hypertriglyceridemic and Prooxidative Effects of Fructose," **American Society of Nutritional Sciences Journal of Nutrition** 132:3370-3382 Nov 2002

[43] Townsend Letter for Doctors, March 1993

[44] Aguilera, A.A., *et al.* (2004). "Effects of fish oil on hypertension, plasma lipids, and tumor necrosis factor-alpha in rats with sucrose-induced metabolic syndrome," **J Nutr Biochem** 2004 Jun; 15(6): 350-7

[45] Ten, S. & Maclaren, N. (2004), "Insulin resistance syndrome in children," **J Clin Endocrinol Metab** 2004 Jun; 89(6): 2526-39

[46] Satoshi Fukuchi (2004). "Role of fatty acid composition in the development of metabolic disorders in sucrose-induced obese rats," **Experimental Biology and Medicine** 229 (6): 486–493

[47] Lombardo, Y.B., *et al.* (1996). "Long-term administration of a sucrose-rich diet to normal rats: relationship between metabolic and hormonal profiles and morphological changes in the endocrine pancreas." **Metabolism** 1996 Dec; 45(12): 1527-32

[48] George A Bray, Samara Joy Nielsen and Barry M Popkin, "Consumption of high-fructose corn syrup in beverages may play a role in the epidemic of obesity." **American Journal of Clinical Nutrition** Vol. 79, No. 4, 537-543, April 2004

[49] Ravi Dhingra, MD, *et al.*, "Soft Drink Consumption and Risk of Developing Cardiometabolic Risk Factors and the Metabolic Syndrome in Middle-Aged Adults in the Community." **Circulation: Journal of the American Heart Association** July 31, 2007

[50] **New Scientist** magazine, Issue 2619, September 4, 2007, page 7

[51] Theresa Waldron, "Sugary Sodas High in Diabetes-Linked Compound," www.healthfinder.gov, a service of the US Department of Health and Human Services

[52] Bantle, John P; Susan K. Raatz, William Thomas and Angeliki Georgopoulos, "Effects of dietary fructose on plasma lipids in healthy subjects," **American Journal of Clinical Nutrition** (November 2000) 72 (5): 1128–1134

[53] Elliott SS, Keim NL, Stern JS, Teff K, Havel PJ (2002), "Fructose, weight gain, and the insulin resistance syndrome," **Am J Clin Nutr** 76 (5): 911–22

[54] Ibid, Bray, George A; Nielsen, Samara Joy; and Popkin, Barry M

[55] Lustig RH (2006), "Childhood obesity: behavioral aberration or biochemical drive? Reinterpreting the First Law of Thermodynamics," **Nature clinical practice. Endocrinology & metabolism,** 2 (8): 447–58

[56] Isganaitis E, Lustig RH (2005), "Fast food, central nervous system insulin resistance, and obesity," **Arterioscler Thromb Vasc Biol** 25 (12): 2451–62

[57] Bray, George A, "How Bad is Fructose," **Am J Clin Nutr** 2007; 86:895– 6

[58] Quoted from Wikipedia, Section on Fructose

[59] Ibid

[60] Teff, KL; Elliott SS, Tschöp M, Kieffer TJ, Rader D, Heiman M, Townsend RR, Keim NL, D'Alessio D, Havel PJ (June 2004), "Dietary fructose reduces circulating insulin and leptin, attenuates postprandial suppression of ghrelin, and increases triglycerides in women," **J Clin Endocrinol Metab** 89 (6): 2963-72

[61] Swan, Norman. ABC Radio National, "The Health Report, The Obesity Epidemic."

[62] Elliott SS, Keim NL, Stern JS, Teff K, Havel PJ (2002), "Fructose, weight gain, and the insulin resistance syndrome, **Am J Clin Nutr** 76 (5): 911–22

[63] Hughes TA, Atchison J, Hazelrig JB, Boshell BR (1989), "Glycemic responses in insulin-dependent diabetic patients: effect of food composition." **Am J Clin Nutr** 49 (4): 658–66

[64] McPherson, JD; Shilton BH, Walton DJ (November 1988), "Role of fructose in glycation and cross-linking of proteins," **Biochemistry** 27 (5): 1901-7

[65] Levi, B; Werman MJ (1998), "Long-term fructose consumption accelerates glycation and several age-related variables in male rats," **J Nutr** 128: 1442-9

[66] Jürgens H, Haass W, Castañeda TR, *et al.* (2005) "Consuming fructose-sweetened beverages increases body adiposity in mice," **Obes Res** 13 (7): 1146–56

[67] Ibid, Bantle JP, *et al*

[68] www.enerex.ca/articles/whey_protein_and_fructose.htp

[69] Melanson, K., *et al* (2006), "Eating Rate and Satiation," Obesity Society (NAASO) 2006 Annual Meeting, October 20-24,Hynes Convention Center, Boston, Massachusetts

[70] Higdon, J. (2003), "Chromium," Linus Pauling Institute, Oregon State University

[71] Buchs, AE; Sasson S, Joost HG, Cerasi E. (1998), "Characterization of GLUT5 domains responsible for fructose transport," **Endocrinology** 139: 827-31

[72] Big Gulp® is a registered trademark of the 7-Eleven company and refers to drinks sold in quantities from 20 to 64 oz.

Chapter 4

[73] DeNoon, Daniel J, "Drink More Diet Soda, Gain More Weight? Overweight Risk Soars by 41% with Each Daily Can of Diet Soft Drink." WebMD Medical News, June 25, 2007

[74] Geoffrey Livesey, "Health potential of polyols as sugar replacers, with emphasis on low glycemic properties," **Nutrition Research Reviews** 2003; 16:163-91

[75] Mendosa, David, "Net Carbs - Can You Really Exclude Sugar Alcohols, Glycerin, Polydextrose, and Fiber?" Published online at www.mendosa.com on February 13, 2004

[76] Rebecca Lian-Loh, Gordon G. Birch, "The metabolism of maltitol in the rat," **British Journal of Nutrition** (1982), 48, 477

[77] Thomas Wolever, "Oral glycerine has a negligible effect on plasma glucose and insulin in normal subjects" **Diabetes** 2005; 51 (Supplement 2): A602

[78] MayAoe Miyoshioka, Yoshiharu Shimomura, and Masashige Suzuki, "Dietary Polydextrose Affects the Large Intestine in Rats," Laboratory of Biochemistry of Exercise and Nutrition, Institute of Health and Sport Sciences, University of Tsukuba, Ibaraki 305, **Japan J. Nutr** 124: 539-547, 1994

[79] Stanford, Duane D., "Coke and Cargill teaming on new drink Sweetener," Atlanta Journal-Constitution, 2007-05-31

[80] Etter, Lauren and McKay, Betsy, " Coke, Cargill Aim For a Shake-up in Sweeteners," **Wall Street Journal**, 2007-05-31

[81] Curi, R, Alvarez M, Bazotte RB, Botion LM, Godoy JL, Bracht A (1986), "Effect of Stevia rabaudiana on glucose tolerance in normal adult humans." **Braz J Med Biol Res** 19 (6): 771-4

[82] Gregersen, S, Jeppesen PB, Holst JJ, Hermansen K (January 2004), "Antihyperglycemic effects of stevioside in type 2 diabetic subjects," **Metabolism** 53 (1): 73-76

[83] The word saccharin has no final "e." The word saccharine, with a final "e" is much older and is an adjective meaning "sugary" – its connection with sugar means the term is used metaphorically, often in a derogative sense, to describe something "unpleasantly over-polite" or "overly sweet." Both words are derived from the Greek word σάκχαρον (sakcharon, German ch sound), which ultimately derives from Sanskrit for sugar, sharkara, which literally means gravel. [Taken from Wikipedia – Section on Saccharin]

[84] The FDA's regulations permit a product to be labeled as "zero calories" if the "food contains less than 5 calories per reference amount customarily consumed and per labeled serving." Code of Federal Regulations, Title 21, Volume 2, Pg. 95 – 101

[85] Michael A. Friedman, Lead Deputy Commissioner for the FDA, "Food Additives Permitted for Direct Addition to Good for Human Consumption; Sucralose," **Federal Register**: 21 CFR Part 172, Docket No. 87F-0086, April 3, 1998

[86] E Ionescu, F Rohner-Jeanrenaud, J Proietto, RW Rivest and B Jeanrenaud, "Taste-induced changes in plasma insulin and glucose turnover in lean and genetically obese rats." **Diabetes** (1988) 37

[87] H. R. Berthoud, E. R. Trimble, E. G. Siegel, D. A. Bereiter and B. Jeanrenaud, "Cephalic-phase insulin secretion in normal and pancreatic islet-transplanted rats." **American Journal of Physiology-Endocrinology and Metabolism** (1980) 238

[88] Sweet'n Low® is manufactured and distributed in the United States by Sugar Foods Corporation. Sweet'N Low sold in the U.S. contains Saccharin and not cyclomate. Sweet'N Low® sold in Canada contains cyclomate and not Saccharin.

[89] Ravi Dhingra, MD; Lisa Sullivan, PhD; Paul F. Jacques, PhD; Thomas J. Wang, MD; Caroline S. Fox, MD; James B. Meigs, MD, MPH; Ralph B. D'Agostino, PhD; J. Michael Gaziano, MD, MPH; Ramachandran S. Vasan, MD, "Soft Drink Consumption and Risk of Developing Cardiometabolic Risk Factors and the Metabolic Syndrome in Middle-Aged Adults in the Community." **Circulation AHA** July 31, 2007, 480-488

[90] Ludwig DS, Peterson KE, Gortmaker SL, "Relation between consumption of sugar-sweetened drinks and childhood obesity: a prospective, observational analysis." **Lancet** 2001; 357: 505-508

[91] Schulze MB, Manson JE, Ludwig DS, Colditz GA, Stampfer MJ, Willett WC, Hu FB, "Sugar-sweetened beverages, weight gain, and incidence of Type 2 Diabetes in young and middle-aged women." **JAMA** 2004; 292:927-934

[92] Winkelmayer WC, Stampfer MJ, Willett WC, Curhan GC, "Habitual caffeine intake and the risk of hypertension in women," **JAMA** 2005; 294: 2330-2335

[93] Ibid, Schulze MB, *et al*

[94] DeNoon, Daniel J, "Drink More Diet Soda, Gain More Weight? Overweight Risk Soars by 41% with Each Daily Can of Diet Soft Drink." WebMD Medical News, June 25, 2007

Chapter 5

[95] Eve van Cauter, "Decreased sleep duration and quality: novel risk factors for obesity and diabetes." A presentation to the 10th European Congress of Endocrinology, May 3-7, 2008, Berlin, Germany, Endocrine Abstracts (2008) 16 PL7. The entire quote follows on the next page.

"Sleep curtailment has become a common behavior in industrialized countries. Simultaneously, the aging of the population is associated with an increased prevalence of sleep disturbances. These trends for shorter sleep duration and poorer sleep quality have developed over the same time period as the dramatic increase in the prevalence of obesity and diabetes. *There is recent evidence to indicate that chronic partial sleep loss and decreased sleep quality may increase the risk of obesity and diabetes* (emphasis added). Studies in healthy volunteers have shown that sleep restriction (4–6 h bedtimes) is associated with an adverse impact on glucose homeostasis. Insulin sensitivity decreases rapidly and markedly without adequate compensation in beta cell function, resulting in an elevated risk of diabetes. Multiple factors appear to mediate this adverse impact of sleep loss, including increased sympathetic nervous activity, decreased brain glucose uptake and elevated evening cortisol levels. Reduced sleep quality, without change in sleep duration, is also associated with an increased risk of diabetes. Indeed, selective suppression of slow-wave sleep, a highly heritable trait, rapidly results in a marked reduction in insulin sensitivity and disposition index. Prospective epidemiologic studies in children and adults are consistent with a role for sleep disturbances in the increased risk of diabetes. Sleep curtailment is also associated with a dysregulation of the neuroendocrine control of appetite. Under conditions of controlled caloric intake and energy expenditure, there is a negative relationship between leptin levels and sleep duration. In a randomized cross-over design study (2 days of 4-h versus 8-h bedtimes), leptin levels were decreased and ghrelin levels increased during the short sleep condition, and the change in the ghrelin to leptin ratio was strongly correlated with increased hunger. Thus, sleep loss may alter the ability of leptin and ghrelin to accurately signal caloric need. Consistent with the laboratory evidence, epidemiologic studies have shown an association between short sleep and higher BMI after controlling for a variety of possible confounders. Taken together, the current evidence suggest that chronic partial sleep curtailment, a novel behavior that appears to have developed with the advent of the 24-h society, and reduced sleep quality may be involved in the current epidemic of obesity and diabetes."

[96] Spiegel K, LeproultR, and Van Cauter E, "Impact of sleep debt on metabolic and endocrine function." **Lancet** (1999) October 23; 354 (9188): 1435-9

[97] Bass J and Turek TW, "Sleepless in America: a pathway to obesity and the metabolic syndrome?" **Arch Intern Med** 2005 Jan 10;165(1):15-6

[98] Jane E Ferrie, PhD; Martin J Shipley, MSC; Francesco P Cappuccio, MD; Eric Brunner, PhD; Michelle A Miller, PhD; Meena Kumari, PhD; Michael G. Marmot, "A Prospective Study of Change in Sleep Duration: Associations with Mortality in the Whitehall II Cohort," **FFPHM Journal SLEEP** Volume 30, Issue 12, pp. 1659-1666, July 08

[99] Ekirch, A Roger, "At Day's Close: Night In Times Past," Orion Publishing House London 2006

[100] Ibid

[101] Trichopoulis D, and Feltcher G, **Internal Medicine**, February 12, 2007; vol 167: pp. 296-301

[102] Parliamentary Office of Science and Technology, "Postnote - The 24 Hour Society." November 2005, Number 250

[103] Bernard, Samuel; Didier Gonze, Branka Čajavec, Hanspeter Herzel, Achim Kramer, "Synchronization-Induced Rhythmicity of Circadian Oscillators in the Suprachiasmatic Nucleus." **PLoS Computational Biology** (2007-04-13) 3 (4)

[104] Edery I, "Circadian rhythms in a nutshell," **Physiol Genomics** 2000 Aug 9; 3(2): 59-74

[105] Sakurai T, Amemiya A, Ishii M, Matsuzaki I, Chemelli RM, Tanaka H, Williams SC, Richardson JA, Kozlowski GP, Wilson S, Arch JR, Buckingham RE, Haynes AC, Carr SA, Annan RS, McNulty DE, Liu WS, Terrett JA, Elshourbagy NA, Bergsma DJ, Yanagisawa M (1998). "Orexins and orexin receptors: a family of hypothalamic neuropeptides and G protein-coupled receptors that regulate feeding behavior." **Cell** 92 (4): 573-85

[106] de Lecea L, Kilduff TS, Peyron C, Gao X, Foye PE, Danielson PE, Fukuhara C, Battenberg EL, Gautvik VT, Bartlett FS, Frankel WN, van den Pol AN, Bloom FE, Gautvik KM, Sutcliffe JG . "The hypocretins: hypothalamus-specific peptides with neuroexcitatory activity." **Proc. Natl. Acad. Sci. U.S.A.** (1998) 95 (1): 322-7

[107] Quoted from the section on "Wakefulness" from the Chapter on Orexin, Wikipedia, 2008

[108] Vanltallie, Theodore B, "Sleep and energy balance: Interactive homeostatic systems." **Metabolism** 2006 Oct; 55 (10 Suppl 2): S30-5

[109] Claude Barnard, "Lecons sur le diabete," Paris, 1877

[110] M Rusek, 1963

[111] RL Hanson

[112] Friedman, M.I., Rawson, N.E. and Tordoff, M.G., "Hepatic signals for control of food intake." (1966) In Bray, G.A. and Ryan, D.H. (editors), **The Genetics and Molecular Biology of Obesity,** LSU Press, Baton Rouge, FL, pp. 318–339

[113] Ji, H and Friedman, MI, "Compensatory hyperphagia after fasting tracks recovery of liver energy status." **Physiol Behav**, (1999) 68, 181–186

[114] Mark I. Friedman, Charles C. Horn and Hong Ji, "Peripheral Signals in the Control of Feeding Behavior." **Chemical Senses** Vol.30 No. Suppl , Oxford University Press 2005

[115] Lavoie, Jean-Marc; Fillion, Yovan; Couturier, Karine; and Corriveau, Pierre; "Evidence that the decrease in liver glycogen is associated with the exercise-induced increase in IGFBP-1." **Journal of Applied Physiology** (May 3, 2002)

[116] Jorgensen, JO; Blum, WF; Horn, N; Moller, N; Moller, J; Ranke, MB; Christiansen, JS; "Insulin-like growth factors (IGF) I and II and IGF binding proteins 1, 2 and 3 during low-dose growth hormone (GH) infusion and sequential euglycemic and hypoglycemic glucose clamps: studies in GH-deficient patients." **Acta-Endocrinol**-(Copenhagen). 1993 Jun; 128(6): 513-20

[117] WS Bullough, and EA Eisa, "The Diurnal Variations In The Tissue Glycogen Content and Their Relation To Mitotic Activity In The Adult Mouse." (1950)

[118] Hansen, J, "Increased breast cancer risk among women who work predominantly at night." **Epidemiology** Vol. 12, January 2001, pp. 74-77

[119] Erren, TC and Piekarski, C, "Does winter darkness in the Arctic protect against cancer? The melatonin hypothesis revisited." **Med Hypotheses**, Vol. 53, July 1999, pp. 1-5

[120] Ravindra T, Lakshmi NK, Ahuja YR, "Melatonin in pathogenesis and therapy of cancer." **Indian J Med Sci** 2006 Dec; 60(12): 523-35

[121] Chantal C, Ruskhsana S, Osborne N, "Melatonin protects primary cultures of rat cortical neurones from NMDA excitotoxicity and hypoxia/ reoxygenation." **Brain Research** Vol 768, Issues 1-2, 12 September 1997, pp. 120-124

[122] Guerrero JM, Reiter RJ, "Melatonin-Immune System Relationships," **Current Topics in Medicinal Chemistry**, Vol 2, Number 2, 1 February 2002, pp. 167-179 (13)

[123] Baydas G, Nedzvetsky VS, Nerush PA, Kirichenko SV, Demchenko HM, Reiter RJ. "A novel role for melatonin: regulation of the expression of cell adhesion molecules in the rat hippocampus and cortex," **Neuroscience Letters** 326(2): 109-12, June 28, 2002

[124] Ibid, Bass J and Turek TW

[125] Carlyle T. Smith, Margaret R. Nixon and Rebecca S. Nader, "Posttraining increases in REM sleep intensity implicate REM sleep in memory processing and provide a biological marker of learning potential." **Learning Memory** 2004 11: 714-719

[126] Ibid, Chepulis, *et al*

[127] Elliot S Valenstein, *"The War of the Soups and the Sparks: The Discovery of Neurotransmitters and the Dispute Over How Nerves Communicate"*

[128] C Smith, "Sleep states and memory processes." **Behavioral Brain Research** 1995 Jul-Aug; 69(1-2): 137-45

[129] Pure unprocessed honey is raw honey that has not been heated above 140 degrees or ultra-filtered after the addition of diatomaceous earth, a process designed to remove all particulate matter from raw honey and lengthen its shelf life.

[130] Leone MV, Chiesa JJ, Marpegan L, Golombek DA. "A time to kill, and a time to heal." **Physiological Mini-Reviews** 2007; 2: 60-69

[131] IGF-1 is a powerful endocrine hormone produced in the liver which stimulates cell growth and multiplication in almost every cell in the human body, especially muscle, cartilage, bone, liver, kidney, skin and lungs. It is a potent inhibitor of the natural process called programed cell death or PCD. When 1GF-1 is inhibited, the process of cellular death continues unabated.

Chapter 6

[132] Cooper, Kenneth C., **Aerobics**. Eldora, Iowa: Prairie Wind, 1968

[133] Adenosine-5'-triphosphate (ATP) is a multifunctional organic compound essential for the intracellular transfer of energy. In other words, ATP transports chemical energy necessary for metabolism within cells.

[134] **No Carbs After 5PM Diet**, Joanna Hall, Publisher. Harper, Thorsons Element, London 2005

[135] Ramussen, BB, Wolfe R R, "Regulation of fatty acid oxidation in skeletal muscle." **Annu Rev Nutr** (1999) 19, 463-484

[136] Wolfe RR, Klein S, Carraro F, Weber J-M, "Role of triglyceride-fatty acid cycle in controlling fat metabolism in humans during and after exercise." **Am J Physiol** (1990) 258, E218-E389

[137] Mermansen L, Hultman E, Saltin B, "Muscle glycogen during prolonged severe exercise." **Acta Physiol Scand** 1967 Oct-Nov, 71(2): 129-39

[138] "Body Fuel Food for Sport," Isabel Walker, Editor, Peak Performance Publishing, London (2005) reprint 2007

[139] Lavoie, Jean-Marc; Fillion, Yovan; Couturier, Karine; and Corriveau, Pierre; "Evidence that the decrease in liver glycogen is associated with the exercise-induced increase in IGFBP-1." **Journal of Applied Physiology** (May 3, 2002)

[140] Cohen, Pinchas, et al. "Insulin-like growth factors (IGFs), IGF receptors, and IGF-binding proteins in primary cultures of prostate epithelial." **Journal of Clinical Endocrinology and Metabolism**, Vol. 73, No. 2, 1991, pp. 401-07

[141] Katz L, De Leon D, Zhao H, Jawad A, "Free and Total Insulin-Like Growth Factor (IGF-1) Levels Decline during Fasting: Relationships with Insulin and IGF-Binding Protein-1." **Journal of Clinical Endocrinology & Metabolism** Vol 87, no 6 2978-1983

[142] Cotterill, AM; Holly, JM; Wass JA; "The regulation of insulin-like growth factor binding protein (IGFBP)-1 during prolonged fasting." **Clinical Endocrinology** (Oxford) 1993 Sep; 39(3): 357-62

[143] WH Busby, DK Snyder and DR Clemmons, "Radioimmunoassay of a 26,000-dalton plasma insulin-like growth factor-binding protein: control by nutritional variables," **Journal of Clinical Endocrinology & Metabolism**, Vol 67, 1225-1230, Copyright © 1988 by Endocrine Society

[144] K Schweighofer, et al, **American Society for Gravitational and Space Biology ASGSB 2006 Abstracts**, "Spaceflight-induced gene expression changes in the mouse: Results from STS-108."

[145] McInnes, Mike and Stuart, **The Hibernation Diet**, Souvenir Press, Ltd, 2006

[146] Ibid, Lavoie, Jean-Marc

[147] Claude Barnard, "Lecons sur le diabete," Paris, 1877

[148] Katz J, McGarry, from "Lecons sur la diabete, The glucose paradox. Is glucose a substrate for liver metabolism?" **J Clin Invest** 1984 December; 74(6): 1901–1909

Chapter 7

[149] "Sport Nutrition for Health and Performance," Melinda Manore, Arizona State University and Janice Thomson, University of New Mexico, Publisher, Human Kinetics, Champaign, IL (2000) p. 43

[150] Kristiansen S, Hargreaves M, Richter EA, "Progressive increase in glucose transport and GLUT-4 in human sarcolemmal vesicles during moderate exercise." **American J Physiol**, March 1997; 272(3 Pt 1): E385-9

[151] S Lancaster, RB Kreider, C Ramsussen, C Kerksick, M Greenwood, A Almada, CP Earnest, "Effect of Honey Supplementation of Glucose, Insulin and Endurance Cycling Performance," The University of Memphis, Exercise & Sport Nutriton Lab, Memphis, TN 38152-3480

[152] Wallis, GA, DA Rowlands, C Shaw, RLPG Jentjens and AE Jeukendrup, "Oxidation of combined ingestion of maltodextrins and fructose during exercise." **Medicine and Science in Sports and Exercise** 37(3): 426-32, 2005

[153] L Roy, PG Jentjiens, Katie Underwood, Juul Achten, Kevin Currell, Christopher H Mann and Asker E Jeudenkrup, "Exogenous carbohydrate oxidation rates are elevated after combined igestion of glucose and fructose during exercise in the heat." **J Appl Physiol**, Mar 2006 100: 807-816

[154] Chepulis L, Starkey N, "The long-term effects of feeding honey compared with sucrose and a sugar-free diet on weight gain, lipid profiles, and DEXA measurements in rats." **Journal of Food Science** (2008) 73 (1) H1-H7

[155] Brooks, GA, "The lactate shuttle during exercise and recovery." **Med Sci Sports Exerc** (1986) 18: 360-368

[156] Ibid, Chepulis L, Starkey N

[157] Wanner H, Gu H, Dorn S, "Nutritional value of floral nectar sources for flight in the parasitoid wasp, Cotesia glomerata." **Physiological Entomology** Volume 31 Issue 2, June 2006, p. 127

[158] **Med Sci Sports Exerc**, Vol 36, No 12, 2107-2111, 2004

[159] Caroline Richmond, "Brian McArdle. One of the last to give his name to an eponymous disease." Obituary in the **British Medical Journal**, August 31, 2002, 325: 497

[160] Adriano Chio, et al, "Severely Increased Risk of Amylotrophic Lateral Sclerosis among Italian Professional Footballers." **Brain Advance Access** Jan 05

[161] Taken from Wikipedia, Section on "Arginine"

[162] American College of Cardiology Annual Scientific Session: Mayo Clinic: March 2008

[163] Ibid

[164] **Overtraining in Sport**, Human Kinetics Publishers, Inc. (1998) Richard B. Kreider, Andrew C. Fry, Mary O'Toole, Editors. Chapter 1, "Overreaching and Overtraining in Endurance Athletes," Mary L O'Toole, PhD

Chapter 8

[165] Ibid, Chepulis L, Starkey N

[166] Yaghoobi N, Al-Waili N, Ghayour-Mobarhan M, Parizadeh SM, Abasalti Z, Yaghoobi Z, Yaghoobi F, Esmaeili H, Kazemi-Bajestani SM, Aghasizadeh R, Saloom KY, Ferns GA, "Natural honey and cardiovascular risk factors; effects on blood glucose, cholesterol, triacylglycerole, CRP, and body weight compared with sucrose." **Scientific World Journal** 2008, April 20; 8: 463-9

[167] Shambaugh P, Worthington V, Herbert JH: Differential effects of honey, sucrose, and fructose on blood sugar levels. **J Manipulative Physiolo Ther** *1990: 13: 322-325*

[168] Ibid, LM Chepulis

[169] Hemoglobin A1c Fact Sheet. Michigan Diabetes Research & Training Center.

[170] Bartol T (December 1, 2000). Comparison of Blood Glucose, HbA1c, and Fructosamine. - a comparison chart that additionally cites: Nathan DM, Singer DE, Hurxthal K, Goodson JD (1984), "The clinical information value of the glycosylated hemoglobin assay". **N. Engl. J. Med**. 310 (6): 341-6

[171] O.P. Agrawal, A. Pachauri, H. Yadav, J. Urmila, H.M. Goswamy, A. Chapperwal, P.S. Bisen, and G.B.K.S. Prasad, "Subjects with Impaired Glucose Tolerance Exhibit a High Degree of Tolerance to Honey," **Journal Of Medicinal Food** 10 (3) 2007, 473–478

[172] Ibid, Prasad, *et al*

[173] Sheard NF, Clark NG, Brand-Miller JC, Franz MJ, Pi-Sunyer FX, Mayer-Davis E, Kulkarni K, Geil P, "Dietary carbohydrate (amount and type) in the prevention and management of diabetes," **Diabetes Care** 2004; 27:2266–2271

[174] Ibid, Busserolles, *et al*

[175] Ibid, LM Chepulis

[176] Ibid

[177] James E. Gangwisch, Steven B. Heymsfield, Bernadette Boden-Albala, Ruud M. Buijs, Felix Kreier, Thomas G. Pickering, Andrew G. Rundle, Gary K. Zammit and Dolores Malaspina, "Short Sleep Duration as a Risk Factor for Hypertension: Analyses of the First National Health and Nutrition Examination Survey," **Hypertension** 2006; 47:833-839

[178] Joseph Bass, MD, PhD, and Fred W. Turek, MD. "Sleepless in America - A Pathway to Obesity and the Metabolic Syndrome?" **Arch Intern Med** VOL 165, JAN 10, 2005

[179] Spiegel K, Leproult R, Van Cauter E. "Impact of sleep debt on metabolic and endocrine function." **Lancet** 1999; 354:1435-1439

[180] Vorona R, Winn MP, Babineau TW, Eng BP, Feldman HR, Ware JC. "Overweight and obese patients in a primary care population report less sleep than patients with a normal body mass index." **Arch Intern Med** 2005; 165:25-30

[181] Findings presented to the British Sleep Society on data taken from 1985-88 with follow up information collected in 1992-93 by teams from University of Warwick and University College London, September 24, 2007

[182] Olofsson, Tobias, PhD, and Vasquez, Alejandra, PhD, "Lactic Acid Bacteria - the Missing Link in Honey's Enigma," Unpublished study presented by the authors at The First International Symposium on Honey and Human Health, January 2008, Sacramento, CA

[183] Rashad UM, Al-Gezawy SM, El-Gezawy E, Azzaz AN, "Honey as topical prophylaxis against radiochemotherapy-induced mucositis in head and neck cancer." **J Laryngol Otol** 2008 May 19:1-6

[184] Motallebnejad M, Akram S, Moghadamnia A, Moulana Z, Omidi S, "The effect of topical application of pure honey on radiation-induced mucositis: a randomized trial." **J Contemp Dent Pract** 2008 Mar 1;9(3):40-7

[185] Al-Waili, Noori S, MD, "Effect of Honey on Antibody Production Against Thymus-Dependent and Thymus-Independent Antigens in Primary and Secondary Immune Responses," **Journal of Medicinal Foods**, 7 (4) 2004, 492–495

[186] Al-Waili, Noori S, MD, PhD, "Short Communication - Effects of Daily Consumption of Honey Solution on Hematological Indices and Blood Levels of Minerals and Enzymes in Normal Individuals." **Journal of Medicinal Foods**, Vol. 6, No 2, 2003

[187] Ibid, Yaghoobi N, *et al*

[188] Al-Waili, Noori S, M.D, PhD; and BONI, NADER S, M.Sc; "Natural Honey Lowers Plasma Prostaglandin Concentrations in Normal Individuals." **Journal of Medicinal Food**, 2003 Summer; 6 (2): 129-33

[189] El-Saleh, Saleh C, "Honey Protects Against Homocysteine Elevation in Rats," **Vascular Disease Pevention**, Volume 3, Number 4, November 2006, pp. 313-318(6)

[190] Bodnoff, S.R., Humphreys, A.G., Lehman, J.C., Diamond, D.M., Rose, G.M. and Meaney, M.J. "Enduring effects of chronic corticosterone treatment on spatial learning, synaptic plasticity, and hippocampal neuropathology in young and mid-aged rats." **J Neurosci** (1995) 15, 61-69

[191] Conrad, C.D., Galea, L.A., Kuroda, Y. and McEwen, B.S. "Chronic stress impairs rat spatial memory on the Y maze, and this effect is blocked by tianeptine pretreatment." **Behav Neurosci**, 1996, 110, 1321-1334

[192] Luine, V.N., Spencer, R.L. and McEwen, B.S., "Effects of chronic corticosterone ingestion on spatial memory performance and hippocampal serotonergic function." **Brain Res** (1993) 616, 65-70

[193] Luine, V., Villegas, M., Martinez, C. and McEwen, B.S., "Repeated stress causes reversible impairments of spatial memory performance." **Brain Res** (1994), 639, 167-170

[194] Mauri, M., Sinforiani, E., Bono, G., Vignati, F., Berselli, M.E., Attanasio, R. and Nappi, G., "Memory impairment in Cushing's disease." **Acta Neurol Scand** (1993) 87, 52-55

[195] Starkman, M.N., Gebarski, S.S., Berent, S. and Schteingart, D.E. "Hippocampal Formation Volume, Memory Dysfunction, and Cortisol Levels in Patients with Cushing's Syndrome." (1992) **Biol Psychiatry** 32, 756-765

[196] Sunil Sharma, MD, FCCP and Rose Franco, MD, FCCP, "Sleep and Its Disorders in Pregnancy." **Wisconsin Medical Journal**, 2004 Volume 103, No 5

[197] Newcomer, J.W., Craft, S., Hershey, T., Askins, K. and Bardgett, M.E., "Glucocorticoid-induced Impairment in Declarative Memory Performance in Adult Humans." **J Neurosci** (1994) 14, 2047-2053

[198] Ibid, Mauri, M., *et al*

[199] Ibid, LM Chepulis, *et al*

[200] Perros P, Deary IJ, Sellar RJ, Best JJ, Frier BM, "Brain abnormalities demonstrated by magnetic resonance imaging in adult IDDM patients with and without a history of recurrent severe hypoglycemia." **Diabetes Care** 1997 June; 20(6): 1013-8

[201] Austin EJ, Deary IJ, "Effects of repeated hypoglycemia on cognitive function: a psychometrically validated reanalysis of the Diabetes Control and Complications Trial data." **Diabetes Care** 1999 August; 22(8): 1273-7

[202] Duval F, Mokrani MC, Monreal-ortiz JA, Fattah S, Champeval C, Schulz P, Macher JP, "Cortisol hypersecretion in unipolar major depression with melancholic and psychotic features: dopaminergic, noradrenergic and thyroid correlates." **Psychoneuroendocrinology** 2006 Aug; 31(7): 876-88

[203] Axelson DA, Doraiswamy PM, McDonald WM, Boyko OB, Tupler LA Patterson LJ, et al., "Hypercortisolaemia and hippocampal changes in depression." **Psychiat Res** 1993 ;47: 163-73

[204] Dinan TG, "Glucocorticoids and the genesis of depressive illness: A psychobiological model." **Br J Psychiatry** 1994; 164:365-71

[205] Rabinach, Arson, "The Human Motor." University California Press, Berkeley and Los Angeles, 1992

[206] Ibid, Dinan TG

[207] Lopez JF, Chalmers D, Little KY, Watson SJ, "Regulation of 5HT1a receptor, glucocorticoid and mineralocorticoid receptor in rat and human hippocampus: Implications for the neurobiology of depression." **Biol Psychiatry** (1998) 43: 547-573

[208] Yudofsky, Stuart C; Hales, Robert E; "The American Psychiatric Publishing Textbook of Neuropsychiatry and Behavioral Neurosciences" 5th (2007) American Psychiatric Pub, Inc.

[209] Ibid, Axelson, *et al*

[210] De Souza, E, "Corticotropin-releasing factor receptors: physiology, pharmacology, biochemistry and role in central nervous system and immune disorders." **Psychoneuroendocrinology** (1995)

[211] Rang HP, Dale MM, "Fructose recycling of NAD from NADH." **Pharamcology** Churchill Livingstone 1991, Edinburgh Chapter 39 pp. 890-1

[212] Al-Waili, Noori S, "Effects of Daily Consumption of Honey Solution on Haematological Indices and Blood Levels of Minerals and Enzymes in Normal Individuals." **Journal Of Medicinal Food** Volume 6, Number 2, 200

[213] Al-Waili, Noori S, Saloom KY, Al-Waili TN, Al-Waili AN, Akmal M, Al-Waili FS, Al-Waili HN, "Influence of various diet regimes on deterioration of hepatic function and haematalogical parameters following carbon tetrachloride: a potential role of natural honey." **Nat Prod Res** 2006 Nov; 20(13): 1258-64

[214] Tarek Swellam, Naoto Miyanaga, Mizuki Onozawa, Kazunori Hattori, Toru Shimazui and Hideyuki Akaza, "Antineoplastic activity of honey in an experimental bladder cancer implantation model: In vivo and in vitro studies." **International Journal of Urology**, Volume 10, Issue 4 (March 2003) pp. 213-219

[215] Sara Caltagirone, Cosmo Rossi, Andreina Poggi, Franco O. Ranelletti, Pier Giorgio Natali, Mauro Brumetti, Framcesco B. Aiello, Mauro Piantelli, "Flavonoids Apigenin and Quercetin Inhibit Melanoma Growth and Metastatic Potential." **Int J Cancer** 2000; 87(4): 595-600

[216] Davis W Lamson, Steven M Plaza, "Mitochondrial Factors in the Pathogenesis of Diabetes" **Alternative Medicine Review** Volume 7, Number 2, 2002, pp. 94-111

[217] M Zakikhani, R Dowling, IG Fantus, N Sonenberg, M Pollack, "Metformin is an AMP Kinase-Dependent Inhibitor for Breast Cancer Cells." **Obstetrical & Gynecological Survey** 62(3):182-183 (March 2007)

[218] The findings relating to the potential use of metformin in cancer treatment were recently confirmed at Texas University and will be presented at the American Society of Clinical Oncology (ASCO) 44th Annual Meeting in a poster discussion by Sao Jiralerspong, MD, PhD, and Anna M. Gonzalez-Angulo, MD, both of M. D. Anderson's Department of Breast Oncology.

[219] Abdul Hannan, Muhammad Barkaat Hussain, Muhammad Usman Arshad, "In Vitro Antibacterial Activity of Pakistani Honey Against Clinical Isolates of Typhoidal Salmonellae."

[220] Al-Waili N, "Intrapulmonary Administration of Natural Honey Solution, Hyperosmolar Dextrose or Hypoosmolar Distill Water on Normal Individuals and Patients with Type-2 Diabetes Mellitus or Hypertension: Their Effects on Blood Glucose Level, Plasma Insulin and C-Peptide, Blood Pressure and Peak Expiratory Flow Rate." **Eur J Med Res** (2003) 8: 295-303

[221] Asadi-Pooya AA, Pnjehshahin MR, Beheshti S, "The antimycobacterial effect of honey: an in vitro study." **Riv Biol** 2003 Sep-Dec; 96(3): 491-5

[222] Iareshko AG, Golenitskii AI, Iareshko VA, Zakharchenko AA, "Effect of flower honey and its products on the M. tuberculosis." **Probl Tuberk** 1978 Mar; (3): 83-4 (Russian)

[223] "Resistant TB from Mexico feared. Strain entering U.S. can't be treated with drugs." WorldNetDaily.com. January 31, 2006

Chapter 9

[224] Quoted from "Honey The Gourmet Medicine." Joe Traynor, Kovak Books 2002, p. 5

[225] Traynor, Joe, "Honey The Gourmet Medicine." Kovak Books 2002

[226] Ibid, p. 11,12

[227] Wittmann S, Mavric E, Barth G, Henle T, "Identification and quantification of methylglyoxal as the dominant antibacterial constituent of Manuka (Leptospermum scoparium) honeys from New Zealand." **Molecular Nutrition and Food Research** 2008 April; 52(4): 483-9

[228] Blair, Shona, PhD, Unpublished data presented by the author at the First International Symposium on Honey and Human Health, January 2008, Sacramento, CA

[229] Ibid, Traynor, p. 34

[230] Advanced glycation end-products (AGEs) can be produced simply by heating sugars with fats or proteins (as in cooking). AGEs may also be formed inside the body through normal metabolism and aging. In hyperglycemia or diabetes, AGE formation can be increased beyond normal levels by oxidative stress.

[231] Theodore Koschinsky, Ci-Jiang He, Tomoko Mitsuhashi, Richard Bucala, Cecilia Liu, Christina Buenting, Kirsten Heitmann, and Helen Vlassara, "Orally absorbed reactive glycation products (glycotoxins): An environmental risk factor in diabetic nephropathy." **Medical Sciences** Vol. 94, pp. 6474 – 6479, June 1997. From the Proceedings of the National Academy of Sciences USA.

[232] Dominiczak MH, "Obesity, glucose intolerance and diabetes and their links to cardiovascular disease. Implications for laboratory medicine." **Clin Chem Lab Med** (2003) 41 (9): 1266–78

[233] Brownlee M, "The pathophysiology of diabetic complications: a unifying mechanism," **Diabetes** (2005) 54 (6): 1615–25

[234] Audrey Riboulet-Chavey, Anne Pierron, Isabelle Durand, Joseph Murdaca, Jean Giudicelli, and Emmanuel Van Obberghen, "Methylglyoxal Impairs the Insulin Signaling Pathways Independently of the Formation of Intracellular Reactive Oxygen Species." **Diabetes** Vol. 55, May 2006

[235] Pfeiffer WF, "A multicultural approach to the patient who has a common cold." **Pediatric Review** 2005; 26(5): 170-175

[236] Department of Child and Adolescent Health. "Cough and Cold Remedies for the Treatment of Acute Respiratory Infections in Young Children." Geneva, Switzerland: World Health Organization; 2001

[237] Ian M. Paul, MD, MSc, Jessica Beiler, MPH, Amyee McMonagle, RN, Michele L. Shaffer, PhD, Laura Duda, MD, Cheston M. Berlin Jr, MD, "Effect of Honey, Dextromethorphan, and No Treatment on Nocturnal Cough and Sleep Quality for Coughing Children and Their Parents." **Arch Pediatr Adolesc Med** 2007; 161(12): 1140-1146

[238] Eva Crane, MSc, PhD, Editor, "Honey A Comprehensive Survey," Crane, Russak & Company, Inc., New York (1975), p. 483. Printed in Great Britain

About the Authors

Mike McInnes, MRPS is the author of **The Hibernation Diet** published in 2006. Mike is a Member of the Royal Pharmaceutical Society of the United Kingdom. He and his wife, Theresa, and his son, Stuart, founded ISO Active in Edinburgh, Scotland in 1997. ISO Active specializes in a nutritional approach to health and exercise.

Mike has spend 12 years researching and refining his knowledge of liver physiology and function that formed the basis for **The Hibernation Diet**. This knowledge base has been expanded in **The Honey Revolution** following Mike's participation as a speaker at The First International Symposium on Honey and Human Health held in Sacramento, CA in January 2008.

Ron Fessenden, MD, MPH is a retired medical doctor. Dr. Fessenden received his MD from the University of Kansas School of Medicine in 1970 and his Masters in Public Health from the University of Hawaii School of Public Health in Hawaii in 1982. For the past two years he has been researching and writing about the health benefits of honey.

Dr. Fessenden is the Co-Chairman for the Committee for the Promotion of Honey and Health, Inc., an international organization committed to communicating the message of honey and health, encouraging research on honey, and establishing quality standards for honey worldwide.

For further information please contact:

ISO Active Ltd.
57-57 South Clerk Street
Edinburgh, Scotland
EH8 9PP

0131 622 6101

Or visit www.isoactive.com or www.hibernationdiet.com

Dr. Fessenden may be contacted at:

WorldClassEmprise, LLC
428 Kent, Haddam, KS 66944
www.worldclassemprise.com

or by email at

info@worldclassemprise.com
www.worldclassemprise.com